WITHDRAWN
FROM THE LIBRARY OF
UNIVERSITY OF ULSTER

Community Matrons:

Caring for people with long-term conditions

D0306667

Note

Healthcare practice and knowledge are constantly changing and developing as new research treatments, procedures, drugs and equipment become available. The authors and publishers have, as far as is possible, taken care to confirm that the information in this book complies with the latest standards of practice and legislation. Where examples have been taken from practice in this book pseudonyms have been used to protect the patients' identity.

Community Matrons:

Caring for people with long-term conditions

Editors

Sue Lillyman and Ann Saxon

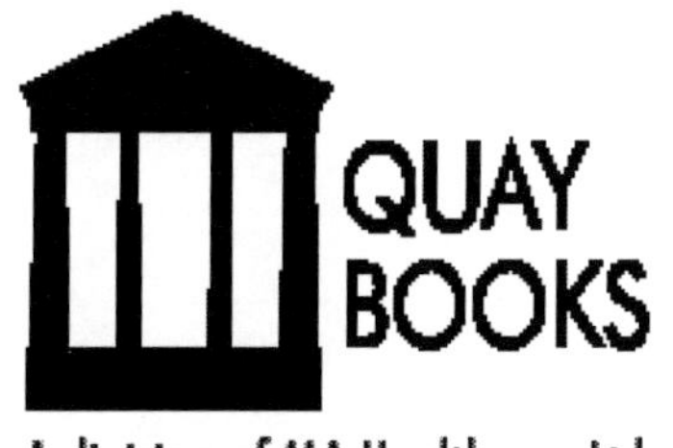

100572683

362.
140941
COM

Quay Books Division, MA Healthcare Ltd, St Jude's Church,
Dulwich Road, London SE24 0PB

British Library Cataloguing-in-Publication Data
A catalogue record is available for this book

© MA Healthcare Limited 2008
ISBN-10: 1-85642-373-5
ISBN-13: 978-1-85642-373-1

All rights reserved. No part of this publication may be reproduced, stored in a retrieval system or transmitted in any form or by any means, electronic, mechanical, photocopying, recording or otherwise, without prior permission from the publishers

Printed by CLE Print Ltd, Media House, Burrel Road, St Ives, PE27 3LE

Contents

Preface

In January 2005 the NHS and Social Care published their document entitled *Supporting People with Long-Term Conditions* (DH 2005). They reported that 17.5 million people in this country currently live with a long-term condition. Although they acknowledge that examples of local excellence are not hard to find, they suggest that we have reached a crucial junction as the number of people living with long-term conditions is set to increase.

The government is committed to improving care for these people by moving away from reactive approach based on acute systems, towards a systematic, patient-centred approach. This approach, they believe, needs to be rooted in the primary care sector, underpinned by communication and new partnerships across the whole health and social care spectrum.

To address these issues set out in the document, this book reviews the role of case manager/community matron as identified by the government. With the introduction of these roles there has been some debate about the title and role this practitioner plays. This book will attempt to identify those practitioners who take on this role, identify the differences between the case manager and community matron and draw on practical experiences from practitioners who have to make difficult decisions out in practice. The book is aimed at any healthcare professional who takes on the role of case manager or community matron.

The book also reviews where the practitioner can move the boundaries forward in their role to achieve the government goals and provide best care for their patients.

We hope that this book will provide information and some practical advice for all professional groups to understand the role of the case manager/community matron and assist those taking up the role to deliver an informed approach to implementing and caring for the person living with a long term condition.

Sue Lillyman and Ann Saxon

Reference

Department of Health (2005) *Supporting People with Long Term Conditions; An NHS and Social Care Model to support local innovation and integration.* London, DH

Acknowledgements

In producing this book we acknowledge our debt of thanks for the support of our colleagues, students, case managers and community matrons who have encouraged us to write such a book.

Introduction

This book is designed to assist the case manager or community matron with issues that they may face within their practice. It is also designed to help other health professionals in secondary and primary care to understand the community matron/case manager's role when working with patients with long-term conditions.

A patient in the latter stages of chronic obstructive pulmonary disease (COPD) identified how the case manager role had helped both him and his wife to cope better with his condition. Previously his only option was to dial 999 and end up in hospital when he felt unwell or needed some advice on his condition. Although the hospital staff could administer antibiotics he found that they were not familiar with his condition and how to manage it, so he was sent home with the same frustrations and questions as he had had before admission.

With a named case manager and specialist practitioner working together to meet his and his family's needs the man felt secure in his own home. He described how all the aids to assist living had been coordinated. A rescue pack with antibiotics for his use had been left so that he could commence treatment when needed. And he was given a phone number to call instead of the ambulance if he felt he needed extra support and advice.

Case manager and community matrons hear many such examples from patients and carers. We hope this book will inspire others to follow the example set by the authors and contributors, as they describe the process they have gone through to deliver that best care for the individual and help them cope with daily life when living with one or more long-term conditions.

Case managers and community matrons in practice have contributed to the production of this book adding a breath and variety of perspectives of the role.

The first chapter reviews the current literature and government documents that relate to this role, identifying the difference between the case manager and community matron. Chapters 2–4 have been written by case managers and identify issues that any manager/matron may be faced with. The final chapters review how the role can be pushed forward and the support systems that these practitioners may access when developing and working with this client group.

Alex Ajao

BSc (Hons) Nursing, BSc (Hons) Community Nursing, RN, PG Cert (Case Management).

Case Manager, Solihull Primary Care Trust

Alex qualified as an enrolled nurse in 1986 at East Birmingham Hospital and in 1992 undertook a BSc (hons) in Nursing at the University of Central England. She then she worked in the community as a district nurse and in 2002 was given the opportunity of visiting Kaiser Permanente in California where she was inspired by the programme of case management. When community matrons were introduced to Solihull in 2005, Alex was instrumental in setting up the service, building on the philosophy of self-management and allowing people to be cared for in their preferred place. After completing the University of Central England's postgraduate certificate in Long-Term Conditions, Alex, with Cecily Harper, formed the West Midlands Community Matron forum aimed as a supportive and learning network for this new role.

Sandra Baines

RN, DN Cert, DPSN.

Respiratory Outreach CNS, Birmingham Eastern and North Primary Care Trust

Sandra commenced her nursing career by completing the orthopaedic certificate in 1977 at the Royal Orthopaedic Hospital in Birmingham before completing her general nursing qualification at East Birmingham Hospital. She remained in orthopaedic and general medicine until she entered district nursing in the late 1980s when she worked in the inner city of Birmingham, for 10 years on the community. Following this, Sandra worked as a tissue viability nurse before taking on the role of discharge planning and care coordinator managing, where she coordinated the discharges for patients who required complex packages of care. Sandra returned to the community as a case manager and has recently moved to respiratory outreach work in the north of Birmingham.

Diane Davies

RN, SN Cert, HV, BSc (Hons), PG Cert (Case Management).

Community Matron

Diane commenced her Registered General Nurse training at St Bartholomew's Hospital, London and qualified in 1988. She became a school nurse for Wolverhampton Health Authority and completed the School Nurse Certificate in 1990. Diane undertook the Health Education Certificate in 1991 and following this became increasingly interested in public health work. Having qualified as a health visitor in 1993, Diane took the lead on a number of health promotion activities, e.g. pioneering the concept of baby massage in Wolverhampton. She completed a BSc Health Studies Degree in 2000 and implemented a number of health visiting service improvement initiatives. In 2005 Diane commenced the role of Case Manager in Wolverhampton City Primary Care Trust, which, through service developments, she has recently evolved into the role of Community Matron.

Cecily Harper

RN, DN cert, PG Cert (Case Management).
Case Manager, Solihull Primary Care Trust
Cecily Harper qualified as an RGN in 1975 at St Bartholomew's Hospital and qualified as a district nurse in 1978 and worked in the North of England before moving to Solihull. Cecily was part of the pilot case management project within Solihull in 2004 and this confirmed her enthusiasm to help develop a model designed to care for people with long-term conditions. When community matrons were introduced to Solihull in 2005 Cecily was instrumental in setting up the service, building on the philosophy of self-management and allowing people to be cared for in their preferred place. After completing the University of Central England's postgraduate certificate in Long-Term Conditions, Cecily, with Alex Ajao, formed the West Midlands Community Matron forum aimed as a supportive and learning network for this new role.

Sarah Knight

RGN, BSc (Hons) Nursing, BSc (Hons) community health with district nursing. PG Cert Ed (Long-term conditions).
Case Manager, Sandwell and West Birmingham NHS Primary Care Trust
Sarah's career in nursing started in 1991 when she commenced a three-year BSc (Hons) course in nursing at what used to be Birmingham Polytechnic. During her time there the title of the institution changed, so she qualified with a 2:1 class degree from the University of Central England. During Sarah's early career, she spent time working on an elderly care ward consolidating her skills, but also developing a strong need to access these patients before they reached the hospital ward. She subsequently started working as a staff nurse within a district nursing team. Sarah soon felt the need to access education to develop her professional career and by 1997 she had completed the BSc (Hons) Community Health with the District Nursing course. Over the years that followed and in between having her children she worked as a district nurse and became a discharge-planning nurse. This was one of the most rewarding parts of her career, accessing patients while in hospital and planning structured discharges for those most complex of patients to ensure they returned and remained at home. After six years within this post Sarah became a case manager. The essence of her role is to prevent avoidable

hospital admissions and to reduce length of stay. Skills she has developed in this role are the advanced nursing skills and non-medical prescribing which are seen as core to this role. Sarah is now in post as the case manager team leader covering a team of about 22 staff ranging from professionals allied to health, nurses, healthcare assistants and administration.

Sue Lillyman

MA (Ed), BSc (Nursing), DPSN, PGCE, RN, RM, RNT.
Senior Lecturer, Birmingham City University
Sue is a qualified nurse and midwife and worked in clinical practice for many years in a variety of hospitals in the West Midlands before entering nurse education in 1989. Recently Sue worked as a volunteer with street boys and helped to set up a medical programme in the Amazonian jungle and has been involved in various medical programmes in the shanty towns of Lima. On returning to the UK, Sue took up a post as senior lecturer at Birmingham City University where she is the route director for the postgraduate certificate in case management of patients with long-term conditions. Sue has had an interest in reflective practice and the improvement of patients care through reflection for many years and has been involved with portfolio development of staff, accreditation of prior learning and professional development. Sue is on the international advisory board of the peer-reviewed journal, *Reflective Practice.* Her work with Reflective Practice UK helps others reach full potential in their workplace through reflection and the development of reflective workplace culture.

Linda Parkes

RN, DPSN, PGCert Case Management of People with Long-Term Conditions.
Case Manager, Sandwell and West Birmingham NHS PCT
Since she qualified as a nurse, Linda's career has evolved around managing the needs of patients with long-term conditions. This pathway began working within a care of the elderly unit and then she became a discharge planning nurse where she also acted as a care manager in the assessment and discharge of patients with complex health needs. Linda is a specialist in continuing health care, acting as a gatekeeper for the provision of resources in the community, including monitoring of services that accurately reflect the changing needs of the patient and carers. As a case manager Linda has continued to hold the responsibilities of a discharge planning nurse and manage the health needs of patients with long-term conditions. Linda currently holds the caseload of approximately 50 patients requiring complex chronic disease management in a densely populated area, where the needs of the clients are diverse and most of the patients have comorbidities that require intense and complex management.

Ann Saxon

MA Education (Health care professionals) PG Dip Education, PG Cert, BSc Health Sciences. RGN, NDN Cert, SEN
Principal Lecturer, University of Wolverhampton

Ann's career started as an Enrolled Nurse at The Birmingham Children's Hospital in 1980 and she converted to a Registered Nurse in 1983. Since then Ann's career has been focused very much in Community as a district nurse and senior nurse managing a range of staff. She moved into education in 1993 following successful completion of her first degree. Ann worked as a Community Tutor at the Birmingham and Solihull College of Nursing and then as a senior Lecturer at UCE Birmingham where she managed the BSc (Hons) Nursing RN course. Ann then moved on to head of division for continuing care post and supported staff in developing innovative ways of delivering education for health professionals. Ann has been involved in Education with colleagues in Finland, Holland and Sweden as part of the ERASMUS programme and with the British Forces in Germany health service. She has also gained a teaching fellowship while at UCE Birmingham for her work in developing discharge planning education.Her current post is at the University of Wolverhampton as Principal Lecturer for postgraduate studies. Ann's interest in case management stems from her work as a community nurse, and her interaction with staff in the hospital setting. She has found it very rewarding to be part of the very first educational programme in the country. It is an important role for nurses to lead and it can have a major impact on the quality of care for patients with long-term conditions and their carers

Sue Talbot

RGN, MSc Advanced Nursing Practice, BSc (Hons), RNT.
Senior Lecturer, University of Wolverhampton

After qualifying in 1976 Sue worked in a variety of clinical areas, including surgical and renal nursing. In 1989 she moved into nurse education, taking responsibility for a number of courses, while undertaking a BSc (Hons) in 1991 and MSc in 1993. In 1996 she became involved in developing the MSc Advancing Clinical Practice and took responsibility for the Role Development Module, for which she is still module leader. With her extensive knowledge of developing the advanced practitioner role, Sue was asked to take responsibility for Developing the Role of the Case Manager as part of the Postgraduate Certificate in Case Management.

Abbreviations

ADL	activities of daily living
COPD	chronic obstructive pulmonary disease
DH	Department of Health
EPP	Expert Patient Programme
FEV	forced expiratory volume
FVC	forced vital capacity ratio
GOLD	Global Initiative for Obstructive Lung Disease
HADS	Hospital Anxiety and Depression Scale
KSF	Knowledge and Skills Framework
LTC	long-term condition
MRC	Medical Research Council
NMC	Nursing and Midwifery Council
NSF	National Service Framework
NYHA	New York Heart Association
OT	occupational therapist
PARR	patients at risk of rehospitalisation
PCT	primary care trust
QALY	quality-adjusted life-years
RCN	Royal College of Nursing
SAP	single assessment process
WHO	World Health Organization
WHOQOL	World Health Organization Quality of Life

CHAPTER 1

Case management and community matron development

Diane Davies

The importance of improving care for people with long-term conditions has become a national priority, as the incidence and subsequently the management costs of care are set to rise (Department of Health 2000). The Department of Health (2004a) heralded the introduction of the new roles of community matron and case manager as one approach to improve the management of individuals with long-term conditions. This included anticipating, coordinating and joining up care of specific high intensity patients, while supporting new ways of working to reduce unplanned hospital admissions and contain costs (Hutt, Rosen & McCauley 2004). Rossi (2003) suggests that the tools of advanced assessment, communication and leadership are key elements of effective case management.

This chapter will outline the new roles and how — through reflection – practitioners can analyse the impact of such new roles.

Analysis of the Case Manager/Community Matron Role

Case management is seen as pivotal in the success of chronic disease management and has been identified as one of the key roles in cost containment strategies developed by the National Health Service (Robinson & Yegian 2004). Dixon et al (2004) note that by focusing on the range of services that need to be in place for chronic disease management and by tailoring the intensity of care provided to match the severity and complexity of care needed, the number of hospital admissions can be reduced. Community matrons and case mangers have been identified as one of the key professionals to implement this new way of working (Goodwin 2006). However, this raises a number of issues relating to the developing case manager role.

Case management is described as a method of proactive care delivery in the community that involves identifying individuals in the population who are at high risk of unplanned admissions, and who have complex and enduring health and social care needs (NatPact 2004). Cesta and Tahan (2003) argue that many health and social care professionals currently undertake case management roles, therefore individuals may be recruited if they have the appropriate skills. However the Department of Health (2006a) state that individuals with complex needs will require input from a community matron defined as:

> *'...a qualified nurse who can provide advanced nursing and clinical care, as well as effective case management'.*
>
> *Department of Health, 2006a*

Robinson (2005) suggests that district nurses or practice nurses are ideally placed to undertake the role of the case manager, as they are already have the clinical assessment skills required for the job, which would negate the need to involve other professionals and thereby reduce duplication. However, O'Dowd (2006) argues that the use of these practitioners will take from the already diminishing pot of nurses in the community and will create gaps in the workforce.

Collaborative Approach

Hutt, Rosen & McCauley (2004) suggest that any discipline with collaboration and communication skills would add a holistic approach to case management. Adams (2005) promotes the successes of case management by working in a team of social workers, therapists and nurses. The Department of Health (2005) acknowledges that the different models of case management could be offered by differing health professionals but tends to emphasise the benefits of a nursing background. Goodwin (2006) suggests that this is short-sighted, that it raises issues about health and social care models of care and undervalues partnership working.

Education Framework

Recently, the Department of Health (2006) *Education Framework for Community Matrons and Case Managers* clarified the specific domains required to undertake the new roles. A distinction between roles needed by community matrons and case managers has been made, notably with the acquisition of advanced assessment skills for the former. This illustrates the importance of the title, although Sands (2007) argues that in future nursing careers would be focused on patient pathways and nursing roles, rather than a title. However, this requires role clarity, which currently appears to be lacking in the development of community matrons and case managers.

Furthermore, the change in title and need to acquire advanced assessment skills and clinical interventions may have increased accountability for some practitioners. Schmitt (2005) suggests that clarity of expressions and boundaries associated with the new role and the meaning ascribed to accomplish these transitions, as a loss or gain of function. This can influence the process of role transition and the degree of role strain experienced. Individual environmental moderators such as personality, social networks, support for learning and availability of resources can also exacerbate or diminish the experience of role strain (Daley 2001).

Development of New Roles

Resistance to change has been identified as a common barrier to role development (Bryar & Griffiths 2003). Bridges (2003) suggests that many attempts to implement change in nursing fail because of the unstructured approach adopted by innovators. O'Dowd (2006) noted that the current transition of this new role into the community had not been smooth.

The different approaches to case management and choice of models, in conjunction with the differing expectations of the case management approach, have led to resistance from other health and social disciplines who do not see a place for the role (Murphy 2004). Anecdotal evidence supports this and highlights the need for a more structured approach. Consistent information-sharing and effective communication are required if individuals, teams and organisations are to undertake the cultural shift of relinquishing traditional roles to accept and support new roles (Hudson & Moore 2006).

Developing New Skills

Evidence suggests that in developing a new role, practitioners are often isolated and lack support, both professionally and educationally (Reade *et al.* 2001). Clegg and Bee (2006) noted that underestimating this can cause practitioners unnecessary anxiety and negatively impacts upon the process of role transition. Senge (2000) suggests that individuals need to be supported in their 'discomfort zone', and by providing a safe environment in which to learn, the psychological process of transition can be nurtured.

Preparation for New Roles

Schmitt (2003) highlights the importance of adequate preparation and educational support to enhance the learning curve for the novice case manager. However, Woodend (2006) notes that the funding restrictions, lack of relevant courses and costs of training impact upon the support given in developing practitioners in a new role.

Mentorship is another key area of support. However, the quality of this may depend on the enthusiasm and availability of appropriate mentors in the workplace.

Furthermore, evidence suggests that the actual provision of education or training for advanced nursing practice has been variable or has not met individual practitioners' learning needs (Thompson & Watson 2003).

Flanagan (2000) advocates commitment and partnership of the practitioner, clinical services and universities to achieve gaps between theory and knowledge and ensure that competency levels of work-based learning are achieved. Learning sets and shadowing have proved to be an effective way to share expertise and build collaboration between established or newly employed case managers and community matrons (Cook 2005). Bowler (2006) advocates clinical supervision as another source of support to underpin evidence-based practice and assist role development.

Importance of the Change Agent

Marketing a service and collaboration with other professionals is seen as essential for role development and effective change management (Castledine & McGee 2003). Marquis and Huston (1996) suggest that the identification of a change agent is a prerequisite for planned change in order to facilitate the process throughout the key stages. Case managers have been identified as such (Evercare 2003) in addition to developing advanced skills with problem solving, decision making and clinical expertise. This may increase the likelihood of change being successful.

Case managers and community matrons need to demonstrate advanced communication skills and creative leadership in promoting collaborative working (NHS Institute for Improvement and Innovation 2005).

Accountability

With the implementation of clinical governance and professional self-regulation, substantial clinical responsibility is being devolved to nurses.

Central to these two concepts is accountability for practice (Gopee 2001). The Nursing and Midwifery Council (2006) provides up-to-date guidelines for accountability. Hickey *et al.* (1996) state that advanced nursing practice is measured against established professional standards for education and expertise, and suggests this assumes that the educational base is uniform throughout the profession for a particular speciality. This raises concerns when considering the varying competency requirements of individual community matrons/case managers currently in post.

Sands (2007) suggests that a more flexible educational base is essential to support depth and breadth of competency achievement. Sawbridge (2005) notes that accountability in role development can further be assisted by the presence of an up-to-date job description, with which staff have been involved and review on an annual basis.

The Department of Health (2004b) *Skills for Health* and *The Knowledge and Skills Framework* (Department of Health 2006) provide a competency framework to assist the process of addressing accountability in developing the role of community matron/case manager. However, research suggests that accountability issues are ongoing, with recent requests from general practitioners for more detail on the boundaries of competent practice and performance, including the effectiveness of the competency assessments of the community matrons (Royal College of General Practitioners 2005). Bird and Morris (2006) argue that overlaps in professional accountability frequently cause confusion regarding authority and responsibility. In addition, feelings of competition result in the creation of barriers to collaboration, necessary to ensure accountable practice.

Conclusion

Limited work has been done to identify the successful components of long-term condition programmes in general and the impact of the role of the community matron specifically (Goodwin 2006). In fact, evidence suggests that the effects of case management approach and community matron interventions varied considerably and were dependant upon the skills and abilities of the case manager providing the care (Gagnon *et al.* 1999). This illustrates the importance of individual practitioners identifying their own learning needs, which are underpinned by adequate and appropriate educational provision, to ensure consistent and safe practice.

References

(all websites accessed 6 March 2008)

Adams R (2005) Case Study: Setting up a case manager team. Unique care development advisor. *Health Service Journal conference, Managing Long-term conditions redesigning services to reduce emergency bed days.* 12th April 2005. London

Bird D, Morris T (2006) Using community matrons to target long-term conditions. *Nursing Times* **102**(23): 19–20

Bowler M (2006) Use of community matrons for care of long-term conditions. *Nursing Times* **102**(33): 31–33

Bridges W (2003) *Managing Transitions: making the most of change* (2nd edn). London, Nicholas Bentley

Bryar R, Griffiths J (2003) *Practice Development in Community Nursing: principles and processes.* London, Arnold Publishers

Castledine G, McGee P (2003) *Advanced Nursing Practice* (2nd edn). Oxford, Blackwell Publishing

Cesta T, Tahan H (2003) *The Case Manager's Survival Guide. Winning strategies for clinical practice* (2nd edn). St Louis, Mosby

Clegg A, Bee A (2006) A model of care for people with long-term conditions. *Journal of Community Nursing.* **20**(9): 13–17

Cook R (2005) *Community Matrons. The Queen's Nursing Institute Briefing Paper.*

Daley B (2001) Learning and professional practice: A study of four professions. *Adult Education Quarterly* **52:** 39–54

Department of Health (2000) *The NHS Plan.* London, DH

Department of Health (2004a) *Skills for Health*, London, DH

Department of Health (2004b) *The NHS Improvement Plan*, London, DH

Department of Health (2005a) *Supporting People with Long-term Conditions: An NHS and Social Care Model to support Local Innovation and Integration.* London, DH

Department of Health (2005b) *The NHS Knowledge and Skills Framework (NHS KSF).* London, DH

Department of Health (2006) *Caring for People with Long-term Conditions: An Education Framework for Community Matrons and Case Managers.* London, DH

Dixon J, Lewis R, Rosen R *et al.* (2004) Can the NHS learn from the US managed care organisations? *British Medical Journal* **326** (24 January): 223–225

Evercare (2003) *Adapting the Evercare Programme for the National Health Service.* (www.natpact.nhs.uk)

Flanagan J (2000) Work-based learning as a means of developing and assessing nursing competence. *Journal of Clinical Nursing* **9**(3): 360–368

Gagnon A, Schein C, McVey L, Bergman H (1999) Randomised control trial of nurse case management of frail older people. *Journal of the American Geriatrics Society* **47:** 1118–1124

Goodwin J (2006) Long-term conditions: how to manage them? *Geriatric Medicine.* Jan 2006: 17–21

Gopee N (2001) Peer review. *British Journal of Nursing* **10**(2): 115–121

Hickey JV, Ouimette R, Venegoni S (1996) *Advanced Practice Nursing: Changing Roles and Clinical Application.* Philadelphia, Lippincott-Raven Publishers

Hudson A, Moore L (2006) A new way of caring for older people in the community. *Nursing Standard* **20**(46): 41–47

Hutt R, Rosen R and McCauley J (2004) *Case managing long-term conditions: What impact does it have on the treatment of older people?* London, The King's Fund, November 2004

Marquis B and Huston C (1996) *Leadership Roles and Management Functions in Nursing: Theory and Practice* (2nd edn) Philadelphia, Lippincott

Murphy E (2004) Case Management and Community Matrons for Long-term conditions. *British Medical Journal* **329:** 1252–1262

National Primary and Care Trust Development Programme (NaTPaCT) (2004) Managing long-term conditions. Cited in Dowse C (2005) Joined-up thinking. *Health Management* 14 Feb: 14–16

NHS Institute for Innovation and Improvement (2005) *Improvement Leaders Guide. Leading Improvement. Personal Organisational Development.* (www.dh.gov.uk/en/Publicationsandstatistics/Publications/PublicationsPolicyAndGuidance/Dh_412701)

Nursing and Midwifery Council (2006) *Accountability A–Z Advice Sheet.* (www.nmc-uk.org)

O'Dowd A (2006) What's the future for community nurses? *Nursing Times* **102**(44): 16–18

Read S, Jones M, Collins K *et al.* (2001) *Exploring New Roles in Practice (ENRIP)* Final report. (www.shef.ac.uk/content/1/c6/01/33/98/enrip.pdf

Robinson F (2005) Chronic disease management. *Community Practitioner* **26**(11): 412

Robinson J and Yegian J (2004) Medical management after managed care. *Health Affairs.* (www.healthaffairs.org)

Rossi P (2003) *Case Management in Health Care* (2nd edn) London, Saunders

Royal College of General Practitioners (2005) *Seven Days.* (www.rcgp.org.uk/default.aspx?page=498) (search archive for June 05 2005)

Sands J (2007) Move to modernise nursing careers. *Independent Nurse* **8**: 21

Sawbridge Y (2005) We must be clear about responsibility. *Independent Nurse* (www.healthcarerepublic.com/news/opinion/576589/clear-responsibility)

Schmitt N (2003) Role transitions for nurses: from caregiver to case manager. Unpublished doctoral dissertation, Michigan Sate University. East Lansing. Cited in Schmitt N (2005) Role transitions from caregiver to case managers, Part one. *Lippincott's Case Management* **10**(6): 294–302

Senge P (2000) *The Dance of Change: Sustaining Momentum in Learning Organisation.* London, Nicholas Bentley

Thompson DR,Watson R (2003) Advanced nursing practice: What is it? (eds) *International Journal of Nursing Practice* **9**(3): 129–130

Woodend K (2006) The role of community matrons in supporting patients with long-term conditions. *Nursing Standard* **20**(20): 51–54

CHAPTER 2

The case manager's challenge

Sandra Baines

'Get Social Services to sort out a ramp so I can get in and out of the flat. Oh, and find me a woman.'

The challenge set by the gentleman — is this the role of a case manager?

This chapter explores the role of a case manager, having regard to current concepts and frameworks for the management of people who live with a long-term condition (LTC).

The Government has identified that the management of a patient diagnosed with a long-term condition should be delivered at three levels (Department of Health (DH) 2005a). These include:

- **Level 1** is aimed at encouraging people to self-manage and self-care. It is estimated that 70–80% of people with a LTC will be in this category
- **Level 2** involves the support of a multidisciplinary team — including general practitioners and specialist nurses — for people with single or multiple conditions, who are at high risk of complications, to assist them to proactively manage their condition
- **Level 3** targets people with highly complex and/or multiple conditions who may have frequent unplanned hospital admissions. It is this minority of people who are to be supported by case managers/ community matrons.

The author of this chapter, working as a community matron, is involved in the second and third level of care provision. This chapter reviews how some of the skills used help the team to promote and coordinate care of this client group.

Choosing an Assessment Model

As the team included an allied health professional they were influenced in considering the role from a broader perspective than just nursing. For this reason, a medical model focus has been avoided and a more holistic approach to the role development occurred. The opportunity to utilise and learn from each other's professional knowledge appears to have been advantageous in expanding the role.

The model proposed by the Government is not prescriptive and leaves opportunities for adaptation by primary care trusts (PCT). It is broadly based on the Kaiser Permanente and Evercare models of disease management developed in the USA. While these models incorporate the principles of case management, it is the reduction in unnecessary admissions and length of stay that appear to be the Government's and PCTs' main focus.

There is debate around the Government's financial commitment to an, as yet, unproved model (Oliver 2005, Roland *et al.* 2005). Roland *et al.* (2005) argue that even without intervention, patients who have high admission rates one year will reduce by 75% the following year. The King's Fund report by Hutt *et al.* (2004:2), has identified only 'weak evidence' supporting the claims of reduced admission rates. However, what has been apparent in case management evaluations has been the level of client satisfaction, reduction in length of hospital stay and improvement in patient outcomes (Hutt *et al.* 2004, Singh 2005, United Health Group 2005). The writer's experience is that this could be attributed to more effective communication and coordination between primary and secondary care and a single point of contact for the patient, family and carers.

Criteria based on total hospital admission rates have been criticised as not being the most reliable source of identifying people who are prone to further admission (Dove *et al.* 2003, Roland *et al.* 2005). Data that identify vulnerable people who use increasing amounts of health and social services resources have been suggested to be better predictors (King's Fund 2005).

Roles of the Case Manager

This chapter will review the differing roles of the case manager in the light of the improvement of patients' care and quality of life.

Dealing with medication compliance

This client group are often on a complex medical regime. The role of the case manager is to monitor that process, review medication regime and prescribe medications. Some patients are left with emergency packs, often containing antibiotics, where the role of the case manager is to assess the abilities of the patient and carer in commencing the medication and education of the patient and care in their use.

Taking a social history

Often there is a history of poor mobility or use of walking aids requiring adaptation to the property inside and outside. There may not be family members living nearby who can support the patient.

In my caseload, one patient was cared for by eight people from health, social services and voluntary services, with no coordination between them. This patient also had two sets of single assessment process documentation and a set of district nursing notes to which no services appeared to pay any regard. There was confusion about how the patient's needs were identified and met.

Taking a psychological history

The geriatric depression scale assessment (Yesavage *et al.* 1983) may be used with this client group. Although there may be no signs of depression, they may identify the feeling of loneliness and losing their self-worth due to the restrictions that the conditions may have made on their quality of life.

Assessment of the client

Some authors suggest that a holistic assessment is not always necessary (Smart 2005). They argue that it exposes patients to unnecessary scrutiny and judgement and suggest that professionals use the knowledge to control people (Foucault 1976). However, it is the writer's belief that a holistic assessment is the cornerstone to effective case management. Consideration must be given to psychological, spiritual, social and financial aspects (James 1992) and an acknowledgment made that disturbances in any of these areas can affect physical health (Ham-Ying 1993). Certainly in one patient's situation, merely addressing his presenting health problems would have ignored factors that were having a significant impact on his health and well-being.

It is advantageous to carry out an advanced physical examination, as part of the assessment, to be able to identify the baseline physical health.

From the initial assessment in one patient it was apparent that the majority of this patient's hospital admissions had been due to falls and that they treated the admissions as 'a holiday' as they were well known to the falls clinic.

Review and coordination of care

One of the principal concepts of case management is the coordination of a person's care and provision of a jointly agreed care plan to identify how their needs are going to be met (DH 2005a, b, c).

From the initial assessment it can be seen that while a number of agencies may be involved and provide care in their areas of speciality, no one agency would have an overall view of all the issues and needs of the patient. It has been suggested that one of the reasons for this may be because staff have insufficient time to assess patients holistically (Smart 2005). Their failure to consider interacting factors may be counterproductive, and result in suboptimal care and increased contact time. In the future we hope that pathways — as identified by the Department of Health (DH 2005a) — will be developed to enable case managers to refer directly to hospital consultants and request investigations, thus avoiding delays in the current process. Our experience has been similar to the Evercare pilot sites. Good working relationships with elderly care consultants are developing (Evercare 2004), but professionals from other specialities have been more circumspect and reluctant to become involved. This may be due to intraprofessional sensitivities (Scholes & Vaughan 2002) and/or confusion about roles and responsibilities (Pearson & Taylor 1996) but is also about developing trust and respect between professionals. This takes time to establish and often, as Scholes and Vaughan (2002) identify, depends on the personality of the postholder.

There were many other examples of how poor communication between agencies was resulting in confusion, repetition of some aspects of care and neglect of others.

In many situations where there are several agencies involved there was a clear need for the case manager to organise case conferences to review patients care however this often requires tact and diplomacy because agencies needed to be challenged and reflect on how care is being delivered and abandon the 'monoprofessional focus' by adopting a multidisciplinary approach to working (Scholes & Vaughan 2002:401). Various writers have identified the factors that teams must consider to enable effective multidisciplinary working. These include:

- Agreed aims and objectives
- Clear identification of roles and responsibilities
- An agreed joint plan of care
- Clear routes of communication
- Clear direction
- An identified coordinator (Sloper 2004, Freeman *et al.* 2000).

Fortunately, a majority of the professionals were willing to work together to improve care. Alder (2005) noted that as case lists became larger, focus moved from proactive to reactive care, so lists should be kept at an optimal number.

While the Government is promoting case management for people with LTC, health and social services authorities are expected to provide increased levels of care within 'existing spending plans' (DH 2005c:5). There is a real risk that case management conducted by community matrons/case managers for LTC in accordance with the Governments initiatives could fail (Whitfield 2004) and health and social services staff become 'scapegoats' due to poor infrastructures and lack of investment (Porter 2005:130).

Patient Education

Patients are often not sure of their own condition and the way to care for themselves. The community matron/case manager is in an ideal position to provide that education to both patients and carers.

Many patients' comorbidities are extremely complex. While the case manager's role includes education of patients and their carers to promote self-care and identify early signs of deterioration (DH 2005a,b) they are expected to be generalist and not specialist practitioners. The case manager may therefore engage specialist practitioners to provide the education required. The case manager needs to be present at education sessions, with the patient's consent, so that information can be reinforced at subsequent visits ensuring that conflicting advice and information is not given — a major factor in non-compliance (Jessiman 1988).

Empowering Patients

Much has been written about empowering patients to make choices about their medical care (DH 2005d, e, Holman & Lorig 2000) and supporting decisions they make even if they do not entirely comply with current professional advice (Metcalf 2005). For patients to be empowered it is essential that they have the necessary knowledge on which to make informed decisions (Kennedy & Rogers 2001). A fundamental role of the case manager is to gain a patient's confidence in order to develop a professional relationship of trust and honesty, thus allowing a patient to identify the gaps in their knowledge. Often in the absence of explicit discussion, professionals can make incorrect assumptions about patients' information needs and preferences (Towle & Godolphin 1999). Cooper (1999) identifies that older people can have long-established, incorrect attitudes and beliefs which negatively affect their ability to manage their disease.

Introduction of Expert Patient Programme (EPP)

The Expert Patient Programme has been developed in response to:

- An acknowledgement that people with long-term conditions are often the people who know best how to manage their illness (DH 2001)
- A move from a paternalistic health model to a partnership approach to healthcare (Thomas 2004).
-

The EPP promotes the concept of patient empowerment and encourages individuals to become involved in decision making, thus improving self-management, increasing control over their own lives and improving self-esteem (DH 2001).

Some patients' experience has shown that an adjustment to the EPP might be an individual patient education programme developed in partnership with the patient. This could ensure patients have the specific individual knowledge to make informed decisions.

Conclusion

Case management for people with LTC provides case managers with a real opportunity to make a difference to the quality of patients' lives. Working in partnership with patients and their families to proactively support them to identify changes in their condition and management of their particular needs is likely to be a real benefit to patient care.

However, if case management is to be successful it must address fundamental issues:

- There needs to be better process at identifying patients who would benefit from the service
- PCTs and the Government need to commit to providing the necessary investment
- Health, social and voluntary services should sign up to a whole system approach to provide the necessary resources to enable people to be cared for either at home or in the local community, thus avoiding unnecessary hospital admissions and a reduced length of stay for any necessary hospitalisation
- A focus on the quality of life needs to be uppermost in case managers' objectives for the patient
- Existing constraints need to be resolved quickly, such as a failure to provide the necessary equipment for advanced health assessments

Case study

The district nurses stated that they had been visiting 'on and off' for six years to dress a patient's leg ulcers. They said the ulcers were normally as a result of the legs becoming grossly oedematous, usually were superficial and healed within a few weeks. They expressed frustration that the patient did not conform to their instructions to go to bed each night so that the legs were elevated, and sitting with their legs raised on a footstool during the day. When the case manager explored these matters with the patient they stated that they had difficulty raising their legs to put them on the stool and experienced severe pain after a short time due to arthritis in both knees. The bed was found to be very low, only some 38 cm from the floor, resulting in the patient having difficulty getting on to and off the bed, and putting them at high risk of falling, so they often slept in the chair.

To address some of these problems, the case manager and the occupational therapist (OT) raised the bed with bed raisers and fitted a bed lever. Experimentation with pillows to support the knees meant that the patient could tolerate elevating their legs. The OT taught the patient how to use a leg raiser to lift his legs onto the stool. The patient has been encouraged to mobilise for short periods and an explanation given that this will promote calf muscle contraction, aid venous return and help reduce leg oedema (Cullum & Roe 1995). Longer-term alternatives were also explored with the OT, including providing a recliner chair.

The case manager took the opportunity to develop links between primary and secondary care. The patient's GP and elderly care consultant discussed the use of low-grade compression to help control oedema. The risk of microvascular disease and peripheral neuropathy due to diabetes and the resultant risk of tissue damage meant that compression therapy could be contraindicated (Moffat & Harper 1997). Consequently, the patient was referred to a vascular consultant for assessment.

- Greater understanding among other professionals of the role of case managers is most important if unnecessary obstacles and delays in implementing case management are to be avoided

- Case managers will need extensive support, and in some cases new professional development and training, to be competent to carry out the range of duties and responsibilities expected of them
- Case managers need to be committed to promoting themselves and the service across both primary and secondary care, thus allaying fears in fellow professionals who may feel threatened by this new role
- In the future the respect and confidence of doctors and consultants in the case manager's role will have to be engendered to open areas that were previously the medics' domain to other professionals

References

(all websites accessed 6 March 2008)

Alder J (2005) What is it like being an advanced primary nurse? *Primary Health Care* **15**(5): 15–17

Cooper J (1999) Teaching patients in post-operative eye care: the demands of day surgery. *Nursing Standard* **13**(32): 42–46

Cullum N, Roe B (1995) *Leg Ulcers Nursing Management: A Research-based Guide.* London, Scutari Press

Department of Health (2001) *The Expert Patient: A new approach to chronic disease management for the 21st century.* London, The Stationery Office

Department of Health (2004a) *Improving chronic disease management.* London, The Stationery Office

Department of Health (2004b) *Chronic disease management: a compendium of information.* London, The Stationery Office

Department of Health (2005a) *Supporting people with long-term conditions: an NHS and social care model to support local innovation and integration.* London, The Stationery Office

Department of Health (2005b) *Supporting people with long-term conditions: liberating the talents of nurses who care for people with long-term conditions.* London, The Stationery Office

Department of Health (2005c) *The National Service Framework for long-term conditions.* London, The Stationery Office

Department of Health (2005d) *Self care – a real choice* London, The Stationery Office

Department of Health (2005e) *Creating a Patient-Led NHS: Delivering the NHS Improvement Plan.* London, The Stationery Office

Dove H, Duncan I, Robb A (2003) A prediction model for targeting low-cost, high-risk members of managed care organisations. *American Journal of Managed Care* **9**(5): 56–69

Evercare (2004) Implementing the Evercare Programme: Interim Report. (www.networks.nhs.uk/39.php)

Foucault T (1976) *The Birth of the Clinic: The Archeology of Medical Perception.* London, Routledge

Freeman M, Miller C, Ross N (2000) The impact of individual philosophies of teamwork on multiprofessional practice and the implications for education. *Journal of International Professional Care* **14**(3): 237–247

Ham-Ying S (1993) Analysis of the concept of holism within the context of nursing. *British*

Journal of Nursing **2**(15): 226–233

Holman H , Lorig K (2000) Patients as partners in managing chronic disease. *British Medical Journal* **320**: 526–527

Hutt R, Rosen R, McCauley J (2004) *Case-managing long-term conditions: what impact does it have in the treatment of older people*? London, The King's Fund

James N (1992) Care = organisation + physical labour + emotional labour. *Sociology of Health and Illness* **14**(4): 488–509

Jessiman D (1988) Causes of non-compliance by patients prescribed eye drops. Cited in Cooper J (1999) Teaching patients in post-operative eye care: the demand for day surgery. *Nursing Standard* **13**(32): 42–46

Kennedy A, Rogers A (2001) Improving self-management skills: a whole systems approach. *British Journal of Nursing* **10**(11): 734–737

King's Fund, New York University, Health Dialog (2005) *Predictive risk project: literature review.* London, The King's Fund

Metcalf J (2005) The management of patients with long-term conditions. *Nursing Standard* **19**(45): 53–60

Moffat C, Harper P (1997) *Leg Ulcers*. Edinburgh: Churchill Livingstone

Oliver D (2005) Interim Report on Evercare illustrates dangers of premature 'good news' briefing. *British Medical Journal* (www.bmj.com/cgi/eletters/330/7486/289)

Pearson A, Taylor B (1996) Gender nursing in colonial Victoria 1840–1870. *International History of Nursing Journal* **2**(1): 25–45

Porter B (2005) Supporting people with long-term conditions. *British Journal of Nursing* **14**(3): 130

Roland M , Dusheiko M , Gravelle H *et al.* (2005) Follow-up of people aged 65 and over with a history of emergency admissions: analysis of routine admission data. *British Medical Journal* **330**(7486): 289–292

Scholes J , Vaughan B (2002) Cross-boundary working: implications for multiprofessional team *Journal of Clinical Nursing* **11**(3): 399–408

CHAPTER 3

Assessment of a patient with a long-term condition, using Pendleton's consultation model

Cecily Harper and Alex Ajao

The notion of nurses undertaking consultations is a relatively new dimension. Consultation models have historically been researched from a GP's perspective (Baird 2004). Sprague (2005) identifies that consultation models should be straightforward, practical and provide guidance that enables advanced nurses to adapt to their new medicalised role.

Although the development of consultation models has been aimed primarily towards doctors, these models should not diminish the nursing essence of caring for patients. Castledine (2003) expresses the need for

Models of Assessment

In the last 50 years, the GP's consultation models have been influenced by:

- **Balint's** (1957) work on the revered function of the GP
- **Byrne & Long** (1976) on identifying doctor's styles
- **Neighbour's** (1987) *The Inner Consultation,* which acknowledges specific areas for 'safe doctoring' viewing the consultation as a vulnerable environment for the doctor, requiring 'safety netting', housekeeping and including building a rapport between patient and GP
- **Kurtz** *et al.* (1998) and **Pendleton** *et al.* (2003), who support the role of the patient as health care provider (Smith 2004).

These models emphasise the importance of arbitration between doctor and patient, both working in partnership, to negotiate patient management plans. The primary focus of the consultation is shifted from the process or task of determining a diagnosis, to patient participation and therapeutic communication.

nurses to be cautious when taking on advanced roles. He urges nurses not to forget the fundamental principles of nursing and reminds us that the interests of patients should be central to nurses' development.

Consultation Models

Duxbury (2002) suggests that the dividing lines between medicine and nursing are becoming hazier and the advanced nurse would benefit from extracting qualities of both nursing and medical models with the emphasis on meaningful dialogue between two people that is goal-directed and patient-centred. McEwan (2004) recognises that consultation models are designed only to provide a framework aimed at guiding practice and improving clinical competence, rather than a strict format.

Pendleton *et al.* (1984) proposed seven tasks that together, taken in any sequence, form a coherent and comprehensive basis for any consultation. These seven tasks are derived from joint perspectives and include the patient's needs, the doctor's aims, the shared desired outcomes and the linking evidence. This allows the patient to feel part of a collaborative

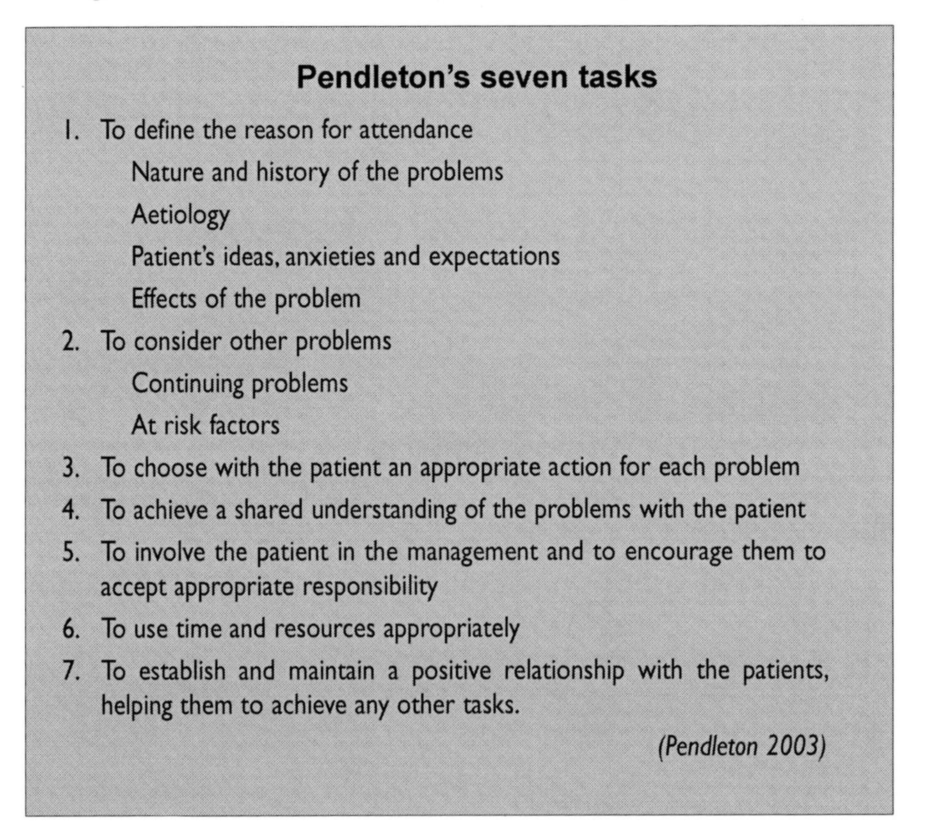
Pendleton's seven tasks

1. To define the reason for attendance
   Nature and history of the problems
   Aetiology
   Patient's ideas, anxieties and expectations
   Effects of the problem
2. To consider other problems
   Continuing problems
   At risk factors
3. To choose with the patient an appropriate action for each problem
4. To achieve a shared understanding of the problems with the patient
5. To involve the patient in the management and to encourage them to accept appropriate responsibility
6. To use time and resources appropriately
7. To establish and maintain a positive relationship with the patients, helping them to achieve any other tasks.

(Pendleton 2003)

process and to build on a practitioner-patient relationship for the future. Pendleton's consultation model (1984) was chosen as a framework for assessing a patient with long-term conditions as it includes self-management, patient empowerment, and relies on partnership working between patient and clinician. These key factors run parallel with the Department of Health (2005) recommendations and guidance for managing people with chronic conditions and were therefore an appropriate model for the community matron to use.

Community matrons, advantageously, can gather information from many sources before visiting the patient, including accessing GP and nursing records (although these should not influence and need to be validated during the patient consultation) (McEvoy 1999).

Single assessment model

The Single Assessment Process (SAP) was introduced as part of the National Service Framework (NSF) for Older People (Department of Health (DH) 2001a) and attempts to ensure that a standardised assessment process is in place across all health and social domains. For the patient, the benefits of SAP are:

- Less duplication and anxiety for the patient
- More involvement in decision-making
- Integrated, seamless and patient-centred care
  (Newson *et al.* 2004, DH 2002).

The NSF (DH 2001a) identified three areas of assessment within SAP:

- Contact
- Overview
- Specialist assessment.

The overview assessment corresponds with the nursing model created by Roper *et al.* (1990) and identifies problems from a patient and clinical perspective, with activities of daily living. The assessment is designed to gather information by observing, measuring and semi-structured questioning (Castledine & McGee 2003).

In theory, the principle of SAP can provide a thorough and effective process, although limitations to its implementation have seen problems between professional groups accepting each other's assessment, and neighbouring trusts developing a wide variety of assessment tools (DH 2004b).

The first task in Pendleton's consultation model (2003) is to define both an understanding of the problem and an understanding of the patient and their perspective. The clinician would establish an initial rapport with the patient and others, described by Neighbour (1987) as '*connecting*'. In contrast Pendleton (2003) does not appear to consider this initial stage of the consultation.

It is highlighted by others that establishing a rapport during the initial stages of the consultation is essential, with the initial greeting having a potential impact on the entire consultation or relationship (Coombe 2003). During consultations, communication skills applied are identical to those in all other nursing situations (Baird 2004) and should aim to facilitate the exchange of ideas and identify concerns, feelings, attitudes and expectations (Smith 2004).

Reflections on a Case Study

General observations start from the moment the community matron meets the patient as these may reveal important diagnostic information.

Case study: Jim

An assessment was arranged for a 78-year-old male patient, Jim (a pseudonym), who had been referred for case management via the district nurses. The GP was fully involved in the referral discussions, promoting interdisciplinary working. Jim's carer was a 74-year-old lady and was a long-standing friend who lived with the patient. She had become increasingly concerned about their situation and ability to cope as Jim's health was progressively deteriorating. He had being admitted to hospital with pneumonia twice in the past four months. The carer herself had a long-standing back 'problem', recognised to be a holistic challenge in itself (Gureje *et al.* 1998).

Observations

On initial observation, Jim was breathless with a cough, an occasional audible wheeze and slight 'purse-lip' breathing. His clothes seemed too big for him, raising suspicion of weight loss, and his house smelt of smoke. Bates (2004) and Douglas *et al.* (2005) offer a systematic overview of the components of history taking and physical examination to focus and guide clinical thinking and reasoning. By recognising the pattern of symptoms, appropriate questions can be asked to determine diagnosis, enabling the consultation to be managed timely and effectively (Douglas *et al.* 2005).

Smith (2004) suggests that observations and history taking supply 60–80% of the diagnostic information, confirming that eliciting information from patients is fundamental to achieving a comprehensive and accurate assessment. Pendleton (2003) supports this and states that the practitioner must understand the disease process and how it can influence patients' perspectives. Douglas *et al.* (2005) affirm that by recognising the pattern of symptoms appropriate questions can be asked to determine diagnosis. The history-taking should include data about physical, biological, psychological and functional status (Royal College of Nursing 1997) that gives rise to the SAP process and requires sophisticated communication (Smith 2004).

History-taking

History taking is a holistic process that involves medical, salutogenic and social factors. Palmer and Kaur (2003) describe *salutogenic* as:

> *'...the ability to cope with life and all its complexities'*.
>
> *Palmer and Kaur (2003)*

This is reliant on personal resources, relationships and a supportive environment. In this case history-taking revealed that Jim was diagnosed with asthma two years previously, seemingly without any proper objective and subjective measurement, and had been prescribed salbutamol and beclomethasone inhalers. His current respiratory symptoms included a chronic cough, producing regular grey-coloured sputum, particularly in the morning, breathlessness even on talking. His carer reported an audible chest wheeze heard on numerous occasions.

Jim had smoked 20 cigarettes a day for approximately 60 years, calculated at a smoking history of 60 pack years. His concerns were his breathlessness and cough, which had not resolved since his second hospital admission four weeks ago. His ability to carry out everyday activities of daily living was affected. Jim felt uncomfortable seeking help from health professionals because of his smoking habit and always being told he must stop. Due to this illness 'experience' his expectations of any increase in functionality were poor. Investigating other problems and risk factors which may include health promotion and addressing issues such as smoking, obesity and social problems are all identified in Pendleton's tasks (2003). His carer was increasingly concerned about Jim's ability to care for himself particularly when her back pain caused her to be 'laid up'.

Physical assessment

After summarising and reflecting with the patient to clarify the situation a general physical examination was undertaken to confirm or refute the possible diagnosis. Jim's blood pressure was within normal limits (Williams *et al.* 2004) and a pulse oximeter was used to evaluate his oxygen saturation status of 94%. Referral for blood gases and other investigations would be needed if the oxygen saturation was below 92% on a stable patient (Bellamy & Booker 2004). Jim had no evidence of peripheral oedema or raised jugular venous pressure to suggest heart failure and/or cor pulmonale. The Medical Research Council (MRC) dyspnoea scale associates levels of mobility with a measurement of the patient's experience and perception of the symptoms of COPD and it can help to determine onset of an exacerbation (McGavin *et al.* 1978). By using the MRC dyspnoea scale, the community matron determined that Jim was stage 4 on the scale as he could not walk further than 100 metres without becoming short of breath.

Respiratory examination includes inspection, palpation, percussion and auscultation (Bates 2004). On inspection, breathing was regular but with effort and it was noted that Jim was using accessory muscles to aid exhalation. Observing and palpating the expansion and symmetry of his chest revealed signs of hyperinflation (barrel chest), and increased antero-posterior diameter and a reduced crico-sternal distance. These signs can often accompany a patient with COPD (Bates 2004). Tactile fremitus of the inferior lobes were slightly decreased in resonance, indicating obstructive sound transmission. Percussion sounded dull in the lower right lung base, suggesting some consolidation that was confirmed on auscultation using the diaphragm of the stethoscope. Auscultation identified the presence of multiple rales or coarse crackles in both lung bases that were not cleared on coughing, along with decreased breath sounds.

By observing Jim's baggy clothes the community matron was led to suspect weight loss. His waist measurement was 75 cm and his Body Mass Index at 18 was calculated to be underweight, which again confirmed that COPD was possible (Bates 2004).

Decision-making

The consultation is a two-way social interaction involving decision making (Tarrant *et al.* 2004) providing a rational choice for both parties. Bakalis and Watson (2004) maintain that the more extensive the nurse's knowledge base is, then the wider selection of prompts are utilised in the deliberation of decision making. They identified that nurses need to be effective decision makers as they often observe rapid deterioration in patients and interpret these events to establish any subsequent action. Macdonald (2005) found that nurse practitioners used four main decision-making concepts in their reasoning strategy:

- Hypothetic-deductive method
- Decision analysis
- Pattern recognition
- Intuition.

The process of recognising patterns intuitively occurs when similarities between a patient's present situation and a comparable patient's past situation are identified. Using both hypothetic-deductive reasoning and pattern matching, the community matron can carefully consider the cues and evaluate the hypotheses to make clinical decisions (Elstein & Schwarz 2002). Having established the most relevant information the community matron may consider a differential diagnosis (Bickley 2003). The patient's previous diagnosis of asthma was unsubstantiated by hard evidence so further investigation was required to confirm an objective diagnosis.

Sharing information

The assessment continued using Pendleton's consultation model (2003), involving agreeing a shared understanding of the problem, examining the appropriate treatment regimes, including lifestyle changes for best management and to improve concordance. Pendleton acknowledges that the patient's agenda has a high priority, although these are often hidden due to fear or uncertainty. Byrne and Long (1976) considered that dysfunctional consultations were mostly due to the clinician failing to understand why the patient had presented. The patient needed a shared understanding of the diagnosis so that he could make an informed decision about further tests and his options for future management.

Diagnosis

The history of symptoms had led the community matron to suspect chronic COPD as a diagnosis. To confirm this, the practitioner needed to elicit objective evidence to support the diagnosis, ensuring the correct treatment was administered. The National Institute for Clinical Excellence (NICE 2004) defines spirometry as being the most definitive diagnostic tool in respiratory disease. Early recognition of the disease, followed by prompt diagnosis and treatment, is a standard required by the Department of Health (2005). COPD is defined as:

'...a chronic, slowly progressive disorder characterised by airflow obstruction, not fully reversible and predominately caused by smoking'

NICE 2004, Bellamy & Booker (2004)

NICE (2004) classifies COPD into three groups by interpreting the results of spirometry testing — mild, moderate and severe. These classifications are deduced by determining the percentage of the predicted forced expiratory volume in one second and forced vital capacity ratio (FEV^1/FVC), with treatment being dependent on the level of disease progression.

A spirometry test established that Jim had an FEV^1 of 1.3 litres and a FVC of 3.1 litres, giving a FEV^1/FVC ratio of 42%, concluding that he had an obstructive abnormality of moderate severity. This gave a diagnosis of moderate COPD (NICE 2004), supported by the patient's history and assessment.

Although NICE (2004) and the Global Initiative for Chronic Obstructive Lung Disease (GOLD 2003) give recommendations for the management and treatment of COPD to promote best practice guidelines, these are recommendations to be used in conjunction with clinical judgement. It is recognised that they do not override the personal responsibilities of health professionals to make appropriate decisions based on the individual circumstance (NICE 2004).

Treatment plans

The community matron shared all the information collected with Jim and his carer so that a joint understanding of the diagnosis, along with the risks and benefits of possible treatments were achieved (Pendleton 2003). Using an approach that values the patients' perspective has been clearly linked with improving concordance with treatment plans (Naidoo & Davy 2005). It acknowledges that both parties may bring a different picture to the consultation with both points of view being equally relevant when deciding on the best management (Weiss & Britten 2003).

Smith (2004) suggests that unless the doctor uses the patient's concepts, ideas and language to fit in with their explanatory models then a number of patients will not remember the key message of the consultation. Shared understanding is achieved when the patient's knowledge and expectations match the likely disease process, management of the problem and its prognosis.

Pendleton's (2003) third consultation task is to enable the patient to choose an appropriate action for each problem. Having shared the options and any implications of treatments the patient must be enabled to decide the actions he wishes to take. Influential factors that will affect his decision-making are recognised as being his personal perception of his quality of life, cultural and ethnic issues, and his contextual view of the disease. The World Health Organization defines quality of life as:

> '*...a subjective evaluation embedded in a specific cultural, social and environmental context*'.
>
> *WHO (1998)*

Quality of life can refer to people's emotional, social and physical well-being, and their ability to function in normal tasks of living (Donald 2003). The difficulty in measuring quality of life is that it is based on subjectivity and influenced by individual values. Laureau *et al.* (1996) state that patients with COPD usually experience gradual degradation in functional status, especially dyspnoea, which will at some point impact on their quality of life. Kennedy (2005) maintains that education around health issues will increase quality of life and longevity. Leplège and Hunt (1997) suggest that the most desirable, patient-centred outcome is improvements within the individual's quality of life and further state that for people with a long-term condition this may be the only achievable outcome.

St George's Respiratory Questionnaire

The St George's Respiratory Questionnaire (Jones *et al.* 1991) is a standardised, reliable, self-completed questionnaire for measuring impaired health and perceived well-being in respiratory disease. Its design allows for comparative measurements of health between patient populations and quantifies changes in health following therapy. The questionnaire includes 56 items across three domains – symptoms, activity and impact – and has been widely used in COPD and asthma studies (Stahl *et al.* 2003). In the complex assessment process undertaken by the community matron, quality of life is addressed by person-centred questions aimed at eliciting subjective responses. This can be achieved by observing mood, thought processes, insight, judgement, memory, attention and calculating abilities throughout the interview (Bates 2004).

Cultural competence

Middleton *et al.* (2005) and Castledine and McGee (2003) maintain that cultural competence is a continuous learning, performing and reflecting cycle. This encourages focusing on oneself as practitioners to become aware of one's own values, beliefs and attitudes. Cultural diversity can be recognised through differences in age, ability, ethnicity, gender, religion and sexuality (Cortis 2003). As cultural beliefs are an integral part of life, it is important that they are central to the consultation process.

Summary of assessment

The assessment led the community matron to identify that Jim was articulate, financially secure and keen to self-manage his condition, thereby maintaining his independence. However, he was a serviceman and had taken up smoking during wartime due to the free supplies. He had admitted to smoking between 10–20 cigarettes a day, having done so for over 50 years. Approximately 90% of COPD cases have a relevant smoking history that is in excess of 15–20 pack years (Bellamy & Booker 2004). NICE (2004) guidelines state that patients should be considered as having COPD if they are over 35 years, have smoked, and have appropriate chronic symptoms of breathlessness, cough and sputum (NICE 2004).

Setting patient goals

Pendleton's (2003) tasks include enabling the patient to manage and accept responsibility of the problem.The community matron discussed goals with Jim and looked at ways in which she could help him to achieve them. These were:

- Going upstairs without having to stop
- Being able to cook again
- Rekindling friendships and go out socially
- Stop smoking.

Hewitt-Taylor (2004) proposes that enabling decision making by patients will challenge the political control or authority that healthcare providers traditionally hold. Palviainen *et al.* (2003) describe power as a matter of authority and control, stating that medicine has traditionally assumed the power to determine what treatment or care individuals should receive, where this should occur and what information they should be given. This approach was based on the concept of expert knowledge being that doctors held the knowledge and power (Kennedy 2003). More recently this has been challenged and there is evidence to support the fact that many patients, particularly those with long-term conditions, are better informed about their condition than healthcare staff (Sobel 1995). There is also evidence that self-care can improve health outcomes (Barlow *et al.*1998) and has been shown to decrease the number of GP consultations by 40% (DH 2005).

Action planning for patients

The community matron proposed a joint action plan that included help with smoking cessation, medication, dietetic and financial review, and referral for pulmonary rehabilitation along with occupational therapy assessment. An application was made for a disabled badge and information on the local carer's association was provided.

Pendleton's consultation model considers other issues, either present problems, problems not yet presented or at risk of developing (Pendleton 2003). At this stage the patient is encouraged to accept responsibility for managing the problems he is faced with. Muncey and Parker (2002) states that the focus of care must concentrate on enabling the person with a long-term condition to live as meaningful and active life as possible. To help enable Jim to take control he was provided with booklets, credible internet sites, contact numbers and information concerning the local group for the expert patient programme (DH 2001b).

The consultation continued with Pendleton's (2003) sixth task of managing time and using it appropriately, although this has been shown to be subjective to the practitioner's experience (Pendleton 2003). In the longer term Naidoo and Day (2005) propose that the length of time a consultation lasts influences patient satisfaction, with longer consultations being favoured. A further point to consider is evidence supporting the fact that patients are less likely to have crises if time is spent on empowerment and self-management (Pendleton 2003).

Multidisciplinary working

Jim was left to absorb the materials and choose how he intended to best manage his condition. It was agreed that the community matron would make the relevant referrals to the appropriate agencies. This final part of the consultation relates to Task 7 where establishing or maintaining a relationship with the patient helps to achieve the other tasks (Pendleton 2003).

Referral to other disciplines involves interagency and interdisciplinary working and using the SAP process is aiding this (DH 2001a).

Integration does pose a threat to '*established ways of working*' (Hudson 2005) who evaluates that '*parity of esteem... acceptance of the judgement of others...and reorientation of professional affinity*' alongside understanding, speed, flexibility and creativity, can enable successful interdisciplinary working. Interdisciplinary care is a shift away from the multidisciplinary care model in that it seeks to blur professional boundaries, requiring trust and tolerance between professional groups and an ability to share responsibility (Hunter *et al.* 1993). Nolan (1995) advocates that this ability to share responsibility is limited by 'professional reductionism' whereby the focus of individual needs is restricted within a given professional paradigm.

The community matron discussed with Jim's GP her consultation findings and the management options. Following NICE (2004) guidelines a long-acting anticholinergic was prescribed providing him with optimal therapy. Emergency antibiotics and steroids as recommended for exacerbations and nicotine replacement therapy were also issued. NICE guideline (2004) state that a patient who is at risk of having an exacerbation of COPD should be given self-management advice that encourages them to respond promptly to the symptoms of an exacerbation.

Shared working continued involving secondary care for chest X-ray results, the physiotherapy for pulmonary rehabilitation, occupational therapy for a stair rail, age concern to aid completion of the disability forms, the council for a disabled mobility badge, the community matron pharmacist to help complete a medication review with the patient and the practice nurse for information on smoking cessation advice. Jim's diet would be reviewed collaboratively and appropriate advice given.

As the role of community matrons becomes more familiar, so will better interdisciplinary working that involves trust and respect for the judgements made in deciding on the patient management options. Kenny (2002) suggests that enabling professions to work collaboratively has little evidence to suggest it reduces bureaucracy and costs. Implementing quality-adjusted life-years (QALYs) estimates, using the league table approach to inform about balancing limited money against greatest health gain, has been criticised for simplifying complex clinical situations (Malek 2003). Using this divisive approach to assess whether an intervention provides value for money has methodological difficulties. Malek (2003) suggests that population health needs and local priorities must be considered when making decisions on health spending (Malek 2003).

Cost benefit of the role of case manager

The case management service has the potential to be cost beneficial in improving clinical outcomes and decreasing the use of NHS resources. Hospitalisation, outpatients and GP consultations could all be reduced as community matrons become more competent, familiar to the system and optimise all treatment options for case-managed patients. COPD is a costly burden, both financially and emotionally, to the lives of the sufferers, their families and to the NHS (DH 2004a).

Jim is working towards his goals, particularly mobility, exercising and smoking cessation and with use of his perching stool he is cooking again. He and his carer have been out socially with help from the local carers' association and they have a purpose to their life again. The carer's back pain has improved, while Jim is considering the Expert Patient Programme (DH 2001a) and awaits an appointment for pulmonary rehabilitation.

Conclusion

Pendleton's consultation model (2003) assumes that consulting is effective if it is patient-centred. However it is difficult to evaluate the relationship between patient-centred models and more traditional versions. The seven tasks are evidence-based and the model is relatively easy to use and it is practical. The limitations include neglecting the practitioner's feelings and the tasks involved could become superficial if beliefs and values are not adaptable. The model needs modifying to truly relate to case management.

To succeed, patients must have a holistic and comprehensive assessment and referral if necessary. The community matron needs to be rational in the decision-making process and include the patient in this process. Positive action has to be forthcoming to improve quality of life for the patient. Awareness of cultural and ethnic issues will help build the trust in the relationship and sharing understanding, management options and information will allow the patient to become empowered and exert self-efficacy to allow success to become apparent.

Interdisciplinary working is to be driven by the benefits to patients across the healthcare system, and though costs–benefits are still inconclusive, there is evidence to support the fact that quality of life costs are improved. The relationship between the value of monetary gains and gains related to health effects such as life years, quality or symptom-free days is a difficult purchasing decision. Case management is presently a committed service and as such patients will be provided with a more personalised and patient centred experience of health provision.

References

(all websites accessed 6 March 2008)

Baird A (2004) *Focus on...the consultation.* (http://journals.cambridge.org/action/displayAbstract?fromPage=online&aid=437222&fulltextTyp)

Bakalis N, Watson R (2005) Nurses' decision-making in clinical practice. *Nursing Standard* **19**(23): 33–39

Balint M (1957) *The Doctor, his Patient and the Illness.* Edinburgh, Churchill Livingstone

Barlow J, Turner A, Wright C (1998) Sharing, caring and learning to take control. *Psychology Health and Medicine* **3**: 387–393

Bates B, Bickley L (2004) *Bates' Guide to Physical Examination and History Taking* (8th edn). London, Lippincott Williams & Wilkins

Bellamy D, Booker R (2004) *Chronic Obstructive Pulmonary Disease in Primary Care* (3rd edn). London, Class Publishing

Byrne P, Long B (1976) *Doctors Talking to Patients.* London, HMSO

Casey G (2001) Oxygen transport and the use of pulse oximetry. *Nursing Standard* **15**(47): 46–53

Castledine G (2003) New nursing roles must retain nursing's principles. *British Journal of Nursing* **12**(21): 3

Castledine G, McGee P (2003) *Advanced Nursing Practice* (2nd edn). Oxford, Blackwell Publishing

Coombe M (2003) Consultation skills. *Registrar Update, MRCGP,* May: 4–6

Cortis J (2003) Managing society's difference and diversity. *Nursing* Standard **18**(14–16): 33–39

Department of Health (2001a) *National framework for older people*. London, DH

Department of Health (2001b) *The Expert Patient: A new approach to chronic disease management for the 21st century.* London, DH

Department of Health (2002) *Introduction to the single assessment process*. London, DH

Department of Health (2004a) *It takes your breath away: the impact of chronic obstructive pulmonary disease*. London, DH

Department of Health (2004b). *West Midlands Regional Single Assessment Group Cross Boundary Working Project.* (www.dh.gov.uk/assetRoot/04/09/86/41/04098641.doc)

Department of Health (2005) *The National Service Framework for Long-term Conditions*. London, DH

Donald A (2003) *What is quality of life?* (http://www.evidence-based-medicine.co.uk)

Douglas G, Nicol F, Robertson C (2005) *Macleod's Clinical Examination* (11th edn). London, Elsevier Churchill Livingstone

Duxbury J (2002) Therapeutic communication and the nurse practitioner. In Walsh M (2005) *Nurse Practitioners: Clinical Skills and Professional Issues*. Edinburgh, Butterworth-Heinemann

Elstein A, Schwarz A (2002) Clinical problem solving and diagnostic decision making: selective review of the cognitive literature. *British Medical Journal* **324:** 729–732

Global Strategy for the Diagnosis, Management and Prevention of Chronic Obstructive Pulmonary Disease (updated2003) *Global Initiative for Chronic Obstructive Lung Disease* (GOLD). (www.goldcopd.com)

Gureje O, Von Korff M, Simon G *et al.*(1998) Persistent pain and well-being. *JAMA* **280** (2): 147–151 (www.jama.ama-assn.org/cgi/conten/abstract/280/2/147)

Hewitt-Taylor J (2004) Challenging the balance of power: patient empowerment. *Nursing Standard* **18**(22): 33–37

Hudson B (2005) Grounds for optimism. *Community Care* 1–7 December 2005: 34–35

Hunter S, Brace S, Buckley G (1993) The interdisciplinary assessment of older people at entry into longer-term institutional care: lessons from the new community care arrangements. *Research, Policy and Planning* **1**(1/2): 2–9

Jones PW, Quirk FH, Baveystock CM (1991) The St George's Respiratory Questionnaire. *Respiratory Medicine* **85**: 25–31

Kennedy I (2003) Patients are experts in their own field. *British Medical Journal* **326** (7402): 1276–1277

Kennedy A (2005) The evidence on quality of life for older people. *Nursing Times* **101**(42): 36–37

Kenny G (2002) Interprofessional working: opportunities and challenges. *Nursing Standard* **17**(6): 33–35

Kurtz S, Silverman, J, Draper, J (1998) *Teaching and Learning Communication Skills in Medicine*. Abingdon, Radcliffe Medical Press

Laureau S, Breslin E, Meek P (1996) Functional Status Instruments: outcome measures in the evaluation of patients with COPD. *Heart and Lung* **25**(3): 212–224

Leplège A, Hunt S (1997) The problem of quality of life in medicine. *JAMA* **278**(1): 47–50

Macdonald J (2005) Higher level practice in community nursing, part 1. *Nursing Standard* **20**(9): 49–51

Malek M (2003) *Implementing QALYs* 3(3). (www.evidence-based-medicine.co.uk)

McEvoy P (1999) Using patients' records as a source of data. *Nursing Standard* **13**(36): 33–36

McEwan A (2004) Consultation and nursing skills: models of consultation. Prescribing Nurse. A supplement to *Practice Nurse* 26–28

McGavin CR, Artvinli M, Naoe H (1978) Dyspnoea, disability and distance walked: Comparison of exercise performance in respiratory disease. *British Medical Journal* **2**: 241–243

Middleton A, Ahmed M, Levene S (2005) Tailoring genetic information and services to clients' culture, knowledge and language level. *Nursing Standard* **20**(2): 52–56

Muncey T, Parker A (2002) *Chronic Disease Management: A Practical Guide*. Basingstoke, Palgrave

Naidoo P, Davy A (2005) *Concepts and Answers for the MRCGP Oral Exam*. Bloxham, Scion Publishing

National Institute for Clinical Excellence (2004) *Management of Chronic Obstructive Pulmonary Disease in Primary and Secondary care*. (www.nice.org.uk/guidance/index.jsp?action=byID&r=true&o=10938)

Newson L, Patel A, Shah R (2004) *Hot Topics for MRCGP and General Practitioners,* 3rd ed. Knutsford, PasTest

Neighbour R (1987) *The Inner Consultation: how to develop an effective and intuitive consulting style*. Lancaster, Kluwer Academic Publishers

Nolan M (1995) Towards an ethos of interdisciplinary practice *British Medical Journal* **311:** 305–307

Palmer D, Kaur S (2003) *Core skills for nurse practitioners*. London, Whurr Publishers

Palviainen P (2003) Do nurses exercise power in basic care situations? *Nursing Ethics* **10**(2): 269–280

Pendleton D, Schofield T, Tate P *et al*. (1984) *The Consultation: an Approach to Learning and Teaching*. Oxford, Oxford University Press

Pendleton D, Schofield T, Tate P *et al*.(2003) *The New Consultation: Developing Doctor-Patient Communication*. Oxford, Oxford University Press

Roper N, Logan W, Tierney A (1990) *The Elements of Nursing* (3rd edn). Edinburgh, Churchill Livingstone

Royal College of Nursing (1997) *The Nursing Older People Assessment Tool*. London, RCN

Smith S (2004) Nurse practitioner consultations: communicating with style and expertise *Primary Health Care* **14**(10): 37–41

Sobel DS (1995) Rethinking medicine: improving health outcomes with cost-effective psychosocial outcomes *Psychosomatic Medicine* **57** (3): 234–244

Sprague D (2005) Consultation skills for nurse practitioners. *Independent Nurse* **20**: 28–29

Stahl E, Jonsson S, Jonsson A *et al*. (2003) Health-related quality of life, utility, and productivity outcomes instruments: ease of completion by subjects with COPD. *Health and Quality of Life Outcomes* **1**(18). (www.hqlo.com/content/1/1/18)

Tarrant C, Stokes T, Colman A (2004) Models of the medical consultation: opportunities and limitations of a game theory perspective. *Quality and Safety in Healthcare 1***3**: 461–466

Weiss M, Britten N (2003) What is concordance? *Pharmaceutical Journal* **271**(7270): 493

Williams B, Poulter NR, Brown MJ *et al*. (2004) The BHS Guidelines Working Party Guidelines for Management of Hypertension: Report of the Fourth Working Party of the British Hypertension Society. *Journal of Human Hypertension* **18**(3): 139–185

WHOQOL World Health Organization Quality Of Life (1998) Development of the WHO Quality of Life Assessment. *Psychological Medicine* **28**(3): 551–558

CHAPTER 4

Models of assessment, diagnosis and management of patients with heart failure

Linda Parkes

This chapter reviews the process of assessment, diagnostics and management of a client undergoing case management. The focus for this chapter will be on the strengths and weaknesses of the model of assessment applied, and an exploration of the effectiveness of the model of clinical reasoning utilised in the management of a patient with a long-term condition. The application of generic and disease-specific quality of life measures used to enhance the assessment and management of patient care will be critically reviewed and will include an illustration of how cultural and ethical awareness can be applied throughout the process. Issues surrounding the effectiveness of interagency and interdisciplinary working will be evaluated, along with consideration of how patient empowerment and self-efficacy can be promoted. Finally, the principles of cost–benefit analysis will be applied to the management of a patient.

The Assessment Process

Huber (2005) describes the assessment process as the gathering of information from relevant sources to better understand the individual needs of the patient. This involves talking to the patient and healthcare providers and includes an in-depth examination of the medical notes to gain an insight into the medical history and current status of the patient. Roper, Logan and Tierney's (1980) activities of daily living can be applied to the assessment process and adapted to include a thorough review of systems. The model is described by Page (1995) as a loose and adaptable framework that can facilitate care through acute and community settings. It is based on a continuum for differing levels of dependence (Page 1995), thus enabling the assessor to focus on patient specific needs to ensure the incorporation of patient goals, including self-management and patient education.

The case manager needs to conduct a comprehensive assessment of the physical, psychological, psychosocial and functional status of the patient, and record the findings as recommended by the Royal College of Nursing (2004). Information and outcomes can be documented using the Single Assessment Process (SAP) (Department of Health (DH) 2001a) which is implemented to ensure assessments are performed using a nationally defined criteria with the overall aim of raising standards (Nazarko 2002). On the whole, it is felt that assessing in this manner achieves a balance between the daily living aspects of care and the biomedical issues to complete this type of complex holistic assessment.

Initial Assessment

Conducting an initial assessment over several visits allows a case manager to see how the patient has used the system. They can also build a rapport to explore the patient's and carer's perceptions of the patient's condition. This assessment process assists us to become aware of the overuse, underuse or potential barriers to the plan of care (Huber 2005). Many patients with chronic illness use the healthcare system inappropriately, so care does not meet the needs of the individual. By addressing problems and taking time to understand patient and provider perspectives, the case manager can develop a goal-directed care plan to meet the needs of the individual whilst achieving satisfactory outcomes for all. Huber (2005) reminds us that gaining acceptance of the plan is essential for success. Its implementation is reliant on presenting evidence-based information, an accurate picture of the current health status and how the plan of care fits into improving the health and function of the patient.

The Single Assessment Process

The Single Assessment Process (SAP) takes a person-centred approach to assessment and enables professionals from different disciplines to contribute. The framework is derived from the good practice described by Nolan and Caldock (1996) and allows elements such as flexibility, appropriateness, balance and incorporation of the views of patients, carers and agencies, and enables these views to be brought together with consideration of the variance of individual situations. SAP allows a platform for professionals to gain the trust of patients by allowing us to recognise them as equal partners in decision making (Nursing and Midwifery Council 2002).

Using SAP to record the information ensures the patient receives appropriate, timely and effective responses to their health and social needs by the effective use of professional resources (DH 2002). By keeping the assessment client-specific and adaptable, every attempt is made to maintain effective good quality care. McKenna (1995) feels this loosely controlled process aids the assessment and with the advanced communication skills of the case manager, enables the more subtle needs of the patient to be highlighted.

Record Keeping

Keeping copies of the assessment documentation in the patient's home is positive in that it allows the patient to reflect on the assessment and plan of care at their convenience, and allows access to all with the patient's consent. However, this method of communication relies heavily on the patient and is thought to become problematic when the patient goes into hospital as the SAP documentation should accompany them at all stages of their journey. The reality is that often the documentation gets left behind or is not kept up to date, which then creates problems in communication and causes ineffective use of time.

Payne *et al.* (2002) describe how methods of transferring information can be improved by using a key person to ensure that assessments and care plans are adequately conveyed. However, the main objective of SAP revolves around patient ownership. Difficulty can also arise in the current paper format used by the case manager in that it creates a barrier between health and social care professionals when attempting to perform joint assessments and planning of patient goals. It has been suggested that an electronic version would be more acceptable and work within the local authority is underway to investigate this option.

Care Pathways

Kelly (2003) believes the model may be enhanced if used in conjunction with a care pathway to offer consistency in the quality of patient care. Locally, such pathways are only a consideration and lessons are being learnt from early implementation sites. Currently the model used is complex and adaptable and relies on the expert communication skills of the professional using the model and the willingness of the patient to explore issues identified during the assessment. Research shows that expert assessment has a direct impact on patient outcomes and the RCN (2004) suggests that the more expert the professional, the more accurate their judgments and predictions will be.

Diagnosis

Due to the complex nature of the patients overseen by the case manager, we are already aware of the diagnosis and long-term condition of the patient, which makes the assessment different to that of a patient with an unknown diagnosis. The case manager may already have prior knowledge of the medical history and treatment regimes of the patient, thus allowing the assessment to be advanced and focus on current symptoms and specific complaints. Dains *et al.* (2003) describe this type of assessment as building on the basic application of a practitioner's knowledge and skills to move from a specific physical finding to a more general diagnosis based on history, physical findings, laboratory and diagnostic tests. Although this enhanced assessment is based on the known diagnosis, caution was taken not to overlook other causes for the experienced problems. Once the evidence is gathered from a variety of sources, the case manager could then narrow down the possibilities; this is otherwise known as diagnostic reasoning (Dains *et al.* 2003). By using this method of assessment, the case manager aims to initiate the best course of treatment with the minimal demand on cost, risk and delay to all involved (Eddy 1996).

Patient History

Dains *et al.* (2003) describe the diagnostic process as commencing with initial evidence being collected through a patient history. For the case manager this includes the gathering of information such as gender, age and occupation to enable the practitioner to place the patient in a risk category and immediately rule out certain diagnoses. Next steps involve the observation of vital signs such as height, weight, temperature, pulse, blood pressure, smoking and alcohol status. Presenting symptoms are explored and goals set to choose the most effective action to gain the health outcome that the patient desires. Dains *et al.* (2003) explain how this step of the decision-making process involves the consideration of benefits outweighing risks, cost-effectiveness and whether the desired outcomes are short- or long-term.

Diagnostic Reasoning

Eddy (1996) goes on to illustrate diagnostic reasoning as a scientific process in which the practitioner suspects the cause of the patient's symptoms and arrives at the correct conclusion to initiate the most efficient and effective course of treatment. From this advanced assessment Dains *et al.* (2003)

confirms that in a patient with a history of heart failure chronic progressive dyspnoea is the most frequent symptom and is often associated with symptoms including oedema, cough, ascites, chest pain and fatigue. These complex problems are ambiguous and presumed to have no standardised treatments. The key to clinical reasoning is knowing what to ask the patient (Dains *et al.* 2003) as these decisions require complex, abstract critical thinking and well-measured judgments.

The case manager and specialist nurse can piece together data from the history, physical examination and laboratory results to differentiate between the diagnostic possibilities and to determine whether emergency intervention is necessary. Nagelkerk (2001) confirms that experienced practitioners develop a process to manage routine and complex decision making efficiently, so the joint working promoted and utilised the appropriate skills to complement and best manage each patient situation.

Collaborative Working

Chronic illness means that concerns can be complicated and change quickly (Huber 2005). Together with the specialist nurse, the case manager educated the patient and carer regarding early warning signs of pertinent health problems. This included information on how to rapidly report concerns to the appropriate health professional thus minimising costly exacerbations.

The aim of this education is to empower the patient to remain in their chosen home environment with support from relevant agencies. This form of education is crucial to the management plan and is backed up by the case manager with documentation to aid communication and patient education to promote self-management. This process of ongoing contact and education between the patient and the case manager is described by Fonarow (1997) as much more effective in managing treatment and preventing admission than that triggered only by symptoms of deterioration.

Evidence-based Practice

Using simple rules of logic to apply evidence from research to a patient's management is defined by Liepzig (1999) as evidence-based practice. It integrates the best research evidence with clinician expertise and the patient's concerns and expectations (Sackett 2000). Once the initial treatment and management plan are established it is not always deemed necessary to manage every problem they experience. Dains *et al.* (2003) believe the knowledge of the patient as a person over time greatly enhances the platform from which the practitioner works to arrive at better clinical judgments. The case manager needs to find a more suitable approach to establish what is needed to be achieved, what relief of a symptom is required or the diagnostic explanation for the symptom. These goals are mutually negotiated to rule out serious conditions and assure patients that their desires and wishes are acknowledged.

Management of Patients with Heart Failure

Redman (2004) reports that one elderly person in 10 suffers from heart failure and the condition is frequently not managed optimally. Blue *et al.* (2001) deem these patients to have a worse prognosis than those with cancer and carry a heavy burden of illness. These findings highlight the importance of advanced continuous assessment and the significance of utilising tools that promote and monitor quality of life issues. Bowling (2001) discusses quality of life as meaning different things to different people. In relation to health, it can be defined in terms of what one has lost or lacks, rather than what one has, and this increases in value and priority with older age. The case manager should attempt to maintain and improve the patient's quality of life by measuring levels of mental, physical, role and social functioning, including some assessment of the patient's level of satisfaction with treatment, outcome and health status. Bowling (2001) agrees that patients' own views are essential in assessments as there are wide discrepancies between patients and professionals ratings. Patient preferences to treatment are considered and care is taken to ensure the patient and carer understand the health risks involved when considering treatment options.

Quality of Life

Although heart disease is common, disease-specific quality of life scales have been poorly developed in relation to cardiovascular diseases (Mayou 1990). Congestive cardiac failure is a chronic and progressively debilitating condition. The heart's failure to maintain adequate output leads to diminished blood flow to the tissues and leads to congestion in circulation. This may lead to shortness of breath upon exertion or lying down and to peripheral oedema, which inevitably affect the patient's activities of daily living.

Quality of life measurements include physical capabilities, emotional status, social interactions, intellectual functioning, economic status and self-perceived health status. Most often the measurement scale used is the New York Heart Association (NYHA) Functional Classification Scale (Criteria

Committee of the New York Heart Association 1964), although data on its reliability and validity is limited. Patients are graded I–IV according to the degree of their physical impairment. However, the scale does not necessarily reflect how a patient feels about their day-to-day level of functioning so it may be necessary to utilise other tools to look at physical, social and emotional well-being to enhance sensitivity.

During assessments, the Medical Research Council dyspnoea scale (MRC 1986) can be used to assess the patient's breathlessness. This tool can be applied in an interviewing scenario and has been used extensively in clinical research as it is shown to correlate strongly with other measures of dyspnoea impairment (Mahler & Harver 1990). Use of the dyspnoea scale is thought to complement the NYHA Scale, best meet a patient's physical needs, and assist in establishing the best management of this symptom.

Heart failure is a progressive condition and a worsening disability that limits patient's activities of daily living so that they become increasingly dependant on carers. Using the Hospital Anxiety and Depression Scale (HADS) (Zigmond & Snaith 1983) equips the case manager to explore a patient's psychological health and refer on to the appropriate professional for advice and support. Positive aspects of the HADS tool include the fact that scale scores are not affected by physical illness and it combines anxiety and depression, so promoting timely and effective measurements with the least distress to the patient. The case manager needs to remember that the tool is primarily used to assess outcomes during hospitalisation and it is unclear how this contrasts with patients in the community.

Management Plan

To complete this ongoing and complex management plan, cultural and ethical beliefs and values need to be explored with the patient and their carer. Although cultural competence in healthcare is well established, it has yet to be fully integrated into healthcare systems (Goode & Suganya 2000). As Nagelkerk (2001) reminds us, practitioners must be culturally sensitive when delivering health care.

The Case Management Service provides care to multicultural groups and attention is paid to variations that may present due to cultural or ethnic origins. These are collected during the initial history taking and information gathering process for the patient. Geissler (1994) believes it can be seen as unrealistic for professionals to have an understanding of the culture of all ethnic or racial groups, as often individuals within a cultural group may not hold the same beliefs.

Professionals need to overcome barriers in cultural communication and be sensitive to individual patients' needs by listening, reinforcing their understanding to the patient and negotiating treatment plans. Ong (1995) reflects that caution needs to be taken to minimise poor health outcomes and reduced satisfaction among patients. The aim of handling these issues in such a sensitive manner is to provide a culturally competent service, increasing knowledge and self-efficacy for the patient as detailed by Smith (2001).

Coordinating Care

The Department of Health (2001b) highlights greater collaboration between agencies as a key priority. SAP relies on a high level of understanding of roles and responsibilities and mutual trust between disciplines. Historically, barriers to effective working are due to mistrust between professionals (NHS Alliance Working Party 2004). Case management strives to diminish these barriers by having a named coordinator for each patient. The assessment and care planning for patients can be compiled using the SAP paperwork shared among all involved.

Langfitt and Meador (2004) find that this method of interagency working prevents unnecessary reassessments and helps to ensure that relevant services are received through the comprehensive and timely completion of records. The interdisciplinary working for patients can be highly effective. The case manager and specialist nurse may conduct joint visits to enhance holistic care and to complement each other's knowledge and use of resources. This has been seen by patients as being highly effective and it considerably reduced duplications. This person-centered service improved the coordination of services and addressed many of the issues associated with disjointed care described in the National Service Framework (DH 2005).

Preventing Admissions to Hospital

The NSF for Older People (DH 2001a) helps to improve leadership and incentives by combining medical and managerial skills to ensure frameworks and resources are in place so that partnerships can function. Billingham (2005) perceives the role of the case manager in emergency situations is to reduce emergency admissions, and for those admitted to reduce the length of stay. For plans to be effective, consideration needs to be given to treatment plans in primary care settings as they rely on low-level technology, stress prevention, encouragement of self-care strategies and open and effective communication between the patient and the case manager (Dains *et al.* 2003). For the management of a patient's care, the case manager needs to strike a balance and coordinate the care the patient receives with the least disruption. Interagency working enables the patient to remain successfully in their own home while receiving treatment from robust domiciliary services and minimal intervention from secondary care.

Patient Self-Management

Most patients have little knowledge of their condition or its treatments. Self-management primarily focuses on optimising treatment regimes. Advice about exercise and diet is rarely given (Redman 2004) but can help heart failure patients take ownership in the management of their condition. Other steps for the more severe condition include patient management of daily weights and monitoring of fluid restrictions. Once established, a patient's self-management can be supplemented by regular contacts from the case manager, frequently by telephone, to detect deterioration and adjust treatment and management of care. The goal of this contact is to decrease hospital admissions and improve quality of life (Cline *et al.* 1998). Riegel *et al.* (2002) confirm in their findings that case management by telephone has found to be effective. However, this type of support is not beneficial to all, for example those with hearing deficiencies. Research by Cline *et al.* (1998) has proven that without this type of intervention, more than half of all such patients are readmitted within six months and half of these hospitalisations are believed to be preventable. The self-management of heart failure patients is considered difficult because early symptoms are subtle and include shortness of breath, increased weight and decreased mental function, the latter of which may only be detected by the carer. The case manager needs to be cautious in advice about the balance of rest and exercise as this information can easily appear contradictory to the patient (Carlson *et al.* 2001).

Advice to Patients with Heart Failure

Due to the multiple comorbidities with related symptoms, patients need advice that is synthesised for all of their illnesses yet specific enough that they will know what to do (Redman 2004). Lack of this advice could lead to poor self-management and non-compliance. Research by Carlson *et al.* (2001) confirms that a large number of patients have little or no self-confidence in their ability to evaluate their actions and this leads to a delay in seeking help until their symptoms clearly indicate that something is happening. However, Redman (2004) suggests self-management could be improved with the use of patient questionnaires to measure the abilities of patients with heart failure to manage their condition. Wakley and Chambers (2005) describe concordance and patient empowerment as key ideals in chronic disease management. Being able to contribute to decisions about their care and understanding their medicines helps the patient to manage many aspects of their treatment, including the use of home oxygen, and to help themselves with carer and professional support.

The Department of Health (2001b) reminds us that up to 50% of people cannot, or do not, take their medications as prescribed. The costs of prescribing these medications is likely to increase as chronic disease management is improved and patients live longer. In 2001, almost 40% of the over-75s took four or more medicines (DH 2001b). It was imperative for the case manager to work with the patient in establishing a good medication review strategy to prevent an important task from becoming an unmanageable burden on clinical time (Wakley & Chambers 2005). Expert Patient Programmes (DH 2001c) play a key part in teaching patients to manage their own long-term conditions and result in a shift in healthcare responsibilities, relieving the pressure on health care costs. Signposting a patient to simple and reliable sources of information can enable them to seek out information at their own convenience. Wakley and Chambers (2005) reinforce the ultimate aim of improving patient outcomes and decreasing stresses on healthcare resources.

Cost of Caring for Patients with Heart Failure

The annual medical cost in the UK for heart failure is currently just over £625 million. Hospital inpatient care is the biggest single health care cost, accounting for approximately 60% of the total cost of heart failure in the UK (British Heart Foundation 2004). Much evidence indicates that patients do not get good value for money (Neumann 2005) and the demand for health care provision will always be greater than the available resources (Evans 1990). The case manager has a duty to reach ethically acceptable solutions in allocating resources and needs to rely on a process of measurement and valuation to strike a balance between the costs of care and benefits to the patient (Williams 1992). Cost–benefit analysis can help determine which healthcare services are most worthwhile. However, Neumann (2005) has found this process to be largely avoided within healthcare, and little attention has been paid to why this is so. Studies such as Eriksen *et al.* (1999) remind us of the high rates of inappropriate hospital admissions that do not result in any significant benefit for the patient and confirm that there is potential for reducing the number of admissions without loss in health benefits. In one case the total bed days of a patient known to case management was reduced by 12 days when compared with the previous 12 months. This comparison supports the wealth of financial and clinical effort used to introduce case management as an effective service.

Conclusion

The successful case management of a patient's long-term condition relies heavily on there being no clear boundaries and the utilisation of various methods to capture information to help ensure an ongoing comprehensive assessment. Many patients may benefit from joint visits as the healthcare professionals can ensure that their roles complement each other's while providing care in a holistic manner to reduce barriers and promote trust. Having one named person to coordinate and direct services is of great benefit to many patients. The assessment is adaptable and this is seen as an important element to maintain good quality effective care. Complexities of using a model of assessment are very dependent on the expertise of the case manager and the expert assessment has a direct impact on practice outcomes. The integrated SAP paperwork can:

- Give a patient a sense of ownership
- Reinforce to them that there is no need to repeat basic information
- Prevented unnecessary reassessment
- Involve a minimum number of professionals.

Goals should be mutually discussed and integrated into a care plan. Clinical goals may be set by the case manager and incorporate the patient's personal goals. Continual monitoring is required as heart failure rates are expected to increase and plans need to be laid down for exacerbations so that these episodes can be managed at home. Throughout the process of assessment the case manager uses clinical and diagnostic reasoning by the process of applying knowledge and experience to the situation to develop a solution. When assuming an exacerbation, the case manager needs to be careful not to miss other causes. The treatment of patients with heart failure is largely symptomatic and many of the management interventions are aimed at improving health-related quality of life. The outcomes for quality of life measures may show improvements in disease-specific and generic quality of life indicators.

An awareness of ethnicity and culture can be applied to the whole process of assessment and management as lack of this could have influenced compliance to treatment and coping strategies. Providing a culturally competent service increased knowledge and self-efficacy for the patient.

The patient and case manager developed a partnership in which the patient was identified as the expert in coping strategies for managing their illness, working with the case manager to provide expertise and knowledge. Some of the most important skills used for this partnership include effective listening, respect, giving timely information and interventions and reflection.

Implementing self-monitoring and acting as a constant contact is the key aspect of self-care and if this is not achieved the health outcomes may be affected. The case manager encompasses the need for an environment where communication between integrated services is vastly improved to enable patients with long-term conditions to stay at home. Evidence to support this improvement may be seen in a patient's behaviour when they begin to use the case manager as a first line of contact for symptoms and medication where previously they would have contacted emergency services. This change in behaviour highlights the capacity of the case manager's role in reducing emergency admissions and bed days.

References

Billingham K (2005) Front line framework. *Nursing Standard* **19**(25): 16–17

Blue L, Lang E, McMurray JJC *et al.* (2001) controlled trial of specialist nurse intervention in heart failure. *British Medical Journal* **323:** 715–718

Bowling A (2001) *Measuring Disease* (2nd edn). Buckingham, Open University Press

British Heart Foundation (2004) *Total Cost of Heart Failure to the NHS.* London, BHF

Carlson B, Riegel B, Moser DK (2001) Self-care abilities of patients with heart failure. *Heart and Lung* **30:** 351–359

Cline CMJ, Israelsson BYA, Willenheimer RB *et al.* (1998) Cost-effective management programme for heart failure reduces hospitalisation. *Heart* **80:** 442–446

Criteria Committee of the New York Heart Association (1964) *Nomenclature and Criteria for Diagnosis of Disease of the Heart and Blood Vessels* (6th edn). MA, Little, Brown and Co

Dains JE Baumann LC, Scheibel P (2003) *Assessment and Clinical Diagnosis in Primary Care.* St Louis, Mosby

Department of Health (2001a) *National Service Framework for Older People.* London, DH

Department of Health (2001b) *Medicines and Older People: Implementing Medicines-related Aspects of the NSF for Older People.* London, DH

Department of Health (2001c) *The Expert Patient – A New Approach to Chronic Disease Management for the 21st Century.* London, DH

Department of Health (2002) *Guidance on the Single Assessment Process for Older People.* London, DH

Department of Health (2005) *The National Service Framework for Long-term Conditions.* London, DH

Eddy DM (1996) *Clinical Decision Making: from Theory to Practice.* Sudbury, Jones and Bartlett.

Eriksen BO, Kristiansen IS, Nord E *et al.* (1999) The cost of inappropriate admissions: a study of health benefits and resource utilization in a department of internal medicine. *Journal of*

International Medicine **246**(4): 379–386

Evans D (1990) *Why Should We Care?* London, Macmillan

Fonarow GC (1997) Impact of a comprehensive heart failure management program on hospital readmission and functional status of patients with advanced heart failure. *Journal of the American Geriatric Association* **30:** 725–732

Geissler EM (1994) *Pocket Guide to Cultural Assessment.* St Louis, Mosby

Goode T, Suganya S (2000) Developing policies to address the healthcare needs of culturally diverse clientele. *Home Health Care Management and Practice.* **12**(5): 49–57

Huber DL (2005) *Disease Management: a guide for case managers.* London, WB Saunders Co Ltd

Kelly D (2003) A commentary on 'an integrated care pathway for the last few days of life'. *International Journal of Palliative Medicine* **9**(1): 39

Langfitt J, Meador K (2004) Want to improve epilepsy care? Ask the patient. *Neurology.* **62**(1): 6–7

Liepzig RM (1999) Evidence in palliative medicine: why, what and where? *Keynote Address Delivered at the American Academy of Hospice and Palliative Medicine.* Utah, Snowbird

Mahler D, Harver A (1990) *Dyspnoea.* New York, Future Publishing

Mayou R (1990) Quality of life in cardiovascular disease. *Psychotherapy and Psychosomatics* 54: 99–109

Medical Research Council (1986) *Questionnaire on Respiratory Symptoms: Instructions to Interviewers.* London, MRC

McKenna H (1995) Nursing skill mix substitutions and quality of care: an exploration of assumptions from research literature. *Journal of Advanced Nursing* **21**(3): 452–459

Nagelkerk J (2001*) Diagnostic Reasoning. Case Analysis in Primary Care Practice.* Philadelphia, WB Saunders Company

Nazarko L (2002) Delayed discharges. The legal implications. *Nursing Management* **9**(1): 22–23

Neumann PJ (2005*) Using Cost-effectiveness Analysis to Improve Health Care: Opportunities and Barriers.* New York, Oxford University Press

NHS Alliance Working Party (2004) The need for coordinated management programmes. *Report of a Joint Working Party of the Royal College of Physicians of London, the Royal College of General Practitioners and the NHS Alliance.* London, NHSAWP.

Nolan M, Caldock K (1996) Assessment: identifying the barriers to good practice. *Health and Social Care in the Community* **4**(2): 77–85

Nursing and Midwifery Council (2002) *Code of Professional Conduct.* London: NMC

Ong L (1995) Doctor–patient communication: a review of the literature. *Social Science and Medicine* **40**(7): 903–918

Page M (1995) Tailoring nursing models to clients' needs: using the Roper, Logan and Tierney model after discharge. *Professional Nurse* **10**(5): 284–288

Payne S, Kerr C, Hawker S *et al.* (2002) The communication of information about older people between health and social care practitioners. *Age and Ageing* **20**(31): 107–117

Redman BK (2004) *Patient Self-Management of Chronic Disease. The Health Care Provider's Challenge.* London, Jones and Bartlett

Riegel B, Carlson B, Kopp Z *et al.* (2002) Effect of a standardized nurse case-management telephone intervention on resource use in patients with chronic heart failure. *Archives of Internal Medicine* **162:** 705–712

Roper N, Logan W, Tierney A (1980) *The Elements of Nursing.* Edinburgh, Chruchill Livingstone

Royal College of Nursing (2004) *Nursing Assessment and Older People*. London, RCN

Sackett DL (2000) *Evidence-based Medicine* (2nd edn). Philadelphia, Churchill Livingstone

Smith LS (2001) Evaluation of an educational intervention to increase cultural competence among registered nurses. *Journal of Cultural Diversity* **5**(4): 138–146

Wakley G, Chambers R (2005) *Chronic Disease Management in Primary Care*. Oxford, Radcliffe Publishing Ltd

Williams A (1992) Cost-effectiveness analysis: is it ethical? *Journal of Medical Ethics* **18**(1): 7–11

Zigmond AS, Snaith RP (1983) The Hospital Anxiety and Depression Scale. *Acta Psychiatrica Scandinavica* **67:** 361–370.

CHAPTER 5

The evolving role of the case manager in the NHS

Sue Talbot

Long-term conditions are those at present that cannot be cured but can be treated and controlled over a long period of time by medication and other therapies (Audit Scotland 2005). The World Health Organization (WHO) (2002) stated that chronic health conditions will be the leading cause of disability by the year 2020 and if not successfully managed will become the most expensive problem for healthcare systems. WHO (2002) described four classifications of long-term conditions:

- Communicable diseases
- Non-communicable diseases
- Ongoing impairments in structure
- Long-term mental health problems.

In the UK, 17.5 million people have a long-term health condition, 45% have more than one condition such as diabetes mellitus, chronic obstructive pulmonary disease and heart disease, they experience a poorer quality of life and sometimes premature death for reasons that are preventable (Department of Health (DH) 2004). Current community services are struggling to provide high quality flexible care for patients with long-term conditions.

In the USA, United Healthcare developed a healthcare programme for vulnerable older people (Evercare), which provided enhanced medical care and coordination of services. This has proved to be successful in reducing readmission to hospital, polypharmacy and calls to GPs. The approach was nurse-led care provided proactively in the patient's home (Kane *et al.* 2003). The UK Department of Health asked United Healthcare to help primary care trusts (PCTs) to plan programmes of care for the frail older person to reduce hospitalisation, based on the Evercare Model. From 2003–2005, United Healthcare carried out a pilot study involving nine primary care trusts, to determine the impact of the Evercare model on the health outcomes of elderly people (Gravelle *et al.* 2006). The pilot study found case management added contact, psychological support, regular monitoring and referral, which had not previously been provided to frail elderly people. It also identified that some nurses had been able to intervene to avoid admission to hospital. Surprisingly, case management had no significant impact on the rates of emergency admissions, bed days or mortality in high-risk groups (Gravelle *et al.* 2006).

Healthcare Systems Approach

Care for many people with long-term conditions has traditionally been reactive, unplanned and episodic, which has resulted in the heavy use of secondary care services (DH 2005a). One of the greatest long-term strategic issues facing the NHS is the burden of meeting ongoing healthcare needs, which is set to increase significantly. Current systems are designed for acute care not chronic care, and as a result patients are not adequately taught and supported in their illnesses. Bodenheimer *et al.* (2002) describe this as a passive uninformed patient interacting with an unprepared practice team. It is no longer appropriate to focus on managing acute episodes within the NHS – there has to be a shift from curative to preventive healthcare, old systems of care must be revised to meet current and future healthcare challenges (Weiss 1998). The political impetus to go with case management is the containment of health and social care costs (Evans *et al.* 2005) and chronic conditions could and should be managed in the primary care setting (DH 2002).

Patient Service Agreement

The Department of Health (2005a) estimates that 5% of individuals with chronic disease account for 42% of hospital bed use. The aim is to reduce the number of emergency bed days by 5% by the year 2008. DH (2004) has identified that long-term conditions in the UK account for 80% of GP consultations and 60% usage of hospital beds. A gap in the provision of healthcare identified there was a need to improve and maintain the health of individuals with long-term conditions, avoiding frequent or lengthy hospital admissions, and this could be undertaken by case management.

Case Management

Case management is a complex concept, for which diverse definitions exist (Slack & McEwen 1999). No case management model will be suitable for all healthcare situations, as each possesses their own strengths and weaknesses to meet different goals (Cudney 2002). Case management extends beyond disease management as it provides social and personal needs (Owen 2006), and provides care for patients with complex needs within three broad categories – hospital, community and hospital/community (Stanton *et al.* 2000). Patients are often elderly, with three or more conditions (DH 2004). Case management has been defined in a variety of ways as:

> '*...the process of planning, coordinating, managing and reviewing the care of an individual*'.
>
> *Hutt et al. (2004:1)*

The term case management is used to cover a number of activities, such as acting as a key worker, broker or procurer of packages for patients to promote independence. To elaborate, the DH (2005a) stated that intensive care management can improve the quality of life and outcomes for these patients, dramatically reducing admissions and enabling patients who are admitted to be discharged home more quickly.

Case management developed as a means to provide cost-effective, high-quality patient care (Reimanis *et al.* 2001). According to Lyon (1993) case management serves two purposes:

- To achieve patient-centred outcomes, which includes linking and coordinating the patient to appropriate services for their needs
- To achieve system-related outcomes of cost containment, data gathering and standardisation of services.

As there is no single model of case management, the term is used to describe a range of approaches to improve the organisation and coordination of services for severe complex health problems (Hutt *et al.* 2004). Beardshaw and Towell (1990) describe three case management frameworks:

- **Brokerage**, in which advocacy is the prominent feature matching the service to individual needs
- **Social entrepreneurship**, which focuses on resource budgetary control to provide packages of care to individuals
- **Extension** of the key worker/care coordinator role, as there is an assumption by members of the multidisciplinary team to arrange deliver and monitor care provided for specific clients

Long (2002) describes two models of case management:

- The **interrogative** model that relies on intense oversight with expected cost reduction

University of Ulster LIBRARY

- An **advocacy** model using brokerage services in the best interests of the patient.

Bodenheimer *et al.* (2002b) describe chronic care as taking place within three overlapping galaxies:

- The entire community with its myriad resources, public and private policies
- The healthcare system
- The provider organisation.

The UK has adopted the NHS Health and Social Care Long-term Conditions Model, adapted from American healthcare models by Evercare and Kaiser Permanente (DH 2005a). The aim of the model is to provide a way of systematic working to deliver improved care that matches patients' needs instead of being delivered in an *ad hoc* manner. The model builds on the Kaiser Permanente triangle. To deliver the care, a new clinical specialist role was to be introduced, that of community matron/case manager (DH 2004).

Defining the Community Matron and Case Manager

New roles develop because of political, social, economic factors and gaps in service provision (Spilsbury & Meyer 2001). In 1997 the government placed the patient at the centre of health service delivery. This led to an increase in the demand for healthcare professionals to take on new roles and new ways of working. The gap in healthcare provision for people with long-term conditions provided opportunities for health and social care professionals to develop and advance their roles within the primary care setting. The *NHS Improvement Plan* (DH 2004) highlighted a need for a new type of clinician for the implementation of case management for people with long-term conditions. This person would often be a nurse who would work with health and social care providers to respond to patients' complex care needs. In 2005 the DH announced that it wanted 3,000 community matrons in post across England and Wales by 2007 to provide case management to caseloads of 50–80 people with long-term conditions. By September 2006 only 366 matrons were in post (Staines 2007). This will have a huge impact and implications for implementing the National Service Framework (NSF) for long-term conditions (DH 2005). The strategic aims for the introduction of community matrons are to:

- Reduce the reliance on hospital care
- Increase range and responsiveness of community services

- Improve the quality of care for people with long-term conditions
- Plan for, predict and prevent crises in care management.

Many health and social care professionals were already acting as case managers in providing care packages.

Case Manager

A case manager is defined as:

> *'...most likely to be a nurse, social worker or healthcare professional who will work with individuals who have a dominant complex single condition but still have intensive needs and whose care requires intensive coordination. Their role will include working with these individuals, their carers and other health and social care professionals to develop a personalised care plan...'.*
>
> *Department of Health (2006:5)*

However, some patients will require intensive complex clinical support from a community matron (DH 2006).

Community Matron

A community matron is:

> *'A nurse who provides advanced clinical nursing care in addition to case management'*
>
> *Department of Health (2006:5)*

Community matrons can come from any branch of nursing. However it is most likely to be from primary care, especially district nurses, who will make the transition as they already have some of the necessary skills and experience to undertake case management. However, as the numbers of district nurses in the UK fell by 5% in 2006 (Vere-Jones 2007), there is possibly a potential shortfall of experienced primary care nurses to provide case management. Primary care trusts (PCTs) are likely to consider experienced hospital nurses (DH 2005, Drennan *et al.* 2005). A systematic literature review, group and key informant interviews were used by Drennan *et al.* (2005) to identify what knowledge and support hospital nurses needed to move into new roles in primary care. The study identified that knowledge was more important than being a primary care trained nurse. No empirical evidence was found on how long the transition period would be needed for a nurse to adapt from a hospital to a community setting. However, nurses who fill these roles because of their care experience would not necessarily have the experience to prepare them for new roles and the transition into them (Schmitt 2005). The Department of Health (2006) suggested that case managers may be appointed without having experience in all of the competencies identified in the education framework, but employers must be willing to support and put systems in place to facilitate, supervise and assess learning in clinical practice.

Role Development

Role theory focuses on the study of people and the roles they occupy. It provides a framework in which to explore interactions and dynamics of the multiple roles an individual occupies at any one time (Handy 1993). Schmitt (2005) cites Biddel's (1979) definition of role theory as a science concerned with the study of behaviours that are characteristics of persons, five basic prepositions underlie the science of role theory:

- Roles consist of patterned behaviours that are characteristics of persons
- Roles are associated with sets of persons who share a common identity
- To some extent persons performing a role are governed by expectations that exist and are shared about normative performance
- Roles persist because of their function and are seen as a perceived necessity
- Roles are learned through socialisation and people find joy or sorrow in performing them

Schmitt (2005) describes two perspectives of role development:

- The **structuralist** approach, which is taking on the objectives and identity of the role
- The **social interactionist** perspective, which views the role as an identity for which the person negotiates. It allows the person moving into the role to bring personal values, goals, meanings and attitudes from previous roles.

Schmitt adds that it is important to consider how role transition affects they way that people change their behaviour in new roles. The impact of any changes to traditional roles and ways of working should be understood by the organisation and its workforce.

According to Colyer (2004) a strong political move in the UK has helped nurses and allied health professionals to move away from the traditional NHS role culture — where people did what their job titles stated — to greater role diversity. When designing new roles these fundamental principles should be considered:

- Assessment of the impact of change — how do the new roles impact on other roles and services?
- The role should takes into account personal, professional development and lifelong learning
- Experience from one post to another should be used and accredited (NHS National Workforce Projects 2005:20).

Case manager roles were developed to coordinate care of complex patients in the community, serving as an advocate and procurers of services for the needy, the underserved and those with complicated needs (Weiss 1998). They serve at the interface between secondary and primary care, health and social care.

The role of the case manager depends not on a specific model but on the right person. Harrell and McCulloch (1986) described numerous problems when developing new roles:

- Role ambiguity
- Title confusion and the legal basis
- Resistance from others
- Lack of authority to be able to carry out the role
- Lack of support to be able carry out the tasks of the role
- Lack of clinical role
- Insufficient research on the role
- Role competition.

A qualitative study by Schmitt (2005) on new roles revealed common themes with healthcare professionals entering the case manager role:

- A lack of insight on entry to what was required within the role
- The lack of resources outside their employment setting to assist them with role mastery.

Role transition from caregiver to case manager can be affected by work settings, organisational structures, performance expectations and professional relationships. Plant (1987) says that when moving from a stable role into a new role individuals will go through an area of uncertainty or 'swampy ground' to reach stability or a 'comfort zone'. In the period of uncertainty the individual will need to develop new skills and knowledge and will try to identify areas of responsibility and new opportunities.

A focus study and data collection survey carried out by Stanton and Dunkin (2002) explored the role of case managers and their expectations within the community setting. They found the role complex because of a limited access to services, and a heavy emphasis on good communication skills. Practice skills needed to be broad so they could span different levels of health prevention along the life continuum. How individuals work in an environment will depend upon the effectiveness of the role in the organisation. Plant (1987:46) identifies ten dimensions of role effectiveness:

- Centrality
- Integration
- Proactivity
- Creativity
- Connections
- Giving and receiving help
- Wider organisational value
- Influence
- Personal growth
- Confronting problems.

These can be applied to the role of the case manager. For example, where centrality of the role is important to the organisation, proactivity will allow the case manager to use initiative within their role and connections relates to collaborative working. In relation to Plant's model, all of these would have high role effectiveness.

Oda (1977) states that success in a new role is not just a matter of expertise, it is about articulating the role and getting colleagues to implement it. Oda's three-phase process of specialised role development can be applied to both community matron and case manager roles:

- Clearly identify the purpose and function of the role
- Implement the role through goal-directed interactions
- Achieve positive recognition and support of the role.

Role Strain

Taking on a new role can cause role strain, which can be attributed to:

- The internal politics of the role

- Ethical dilemmas
- Lack of clarity about the role
- Professional boundaries associated with the role.

These may be caused by the individual's personality, self-confidence, self-identity and locus of control. They may also be compounded by a lack of support for learning and poor social networks. Individuals can reduce role strain by seeking out more information about the role; working to gain or enhance specific skills required by the role and by seeking to change behavioural expectations of the role.

Competencies and Education for Case Management

To meet the needs and demands in caring for an expanding population of people with long-term conditions new ways of training and education should be considered (Pruitt & Epping-Jordan 2005). Taylor (1999) and Zander (2002) state an advanced level of education and practice is required for case management. Taylor (1999) elaborated that those case managers with advanced degrees concentrated as a primary focus on patient/family education, problem identification, resolution and evaluation, while those without concentrated on technical tasks and discharge planning. Stanton *et al.* (2005) disagree, stating that not all case managers need a graduate degree or to work at an advanced level to provide nursing care in case management. They identified two levels of practice – basic and advanced – differentiated by competency in clinical practice, educational level and research responsibilities.

Basic case management provides:

- Physical and psychological care
- Collaboration with the multidisciplinary team
- Education
- Supervision of care plans
- Quality control and prevents the fragmentation of care.

Advanced practice is all of these plus disease management and population-based care management. A small qualitative study using focus group interviews by Williamson *et al.* (2005) identified the need for further research to evaluate the impact of a masters degree on patients, service delivery and the organisation.

Many authors have tried to identify the roles and competencies of case managers (see *Table 5.1*).

Table 5.1 Roles of the case manager

Author	Roles
Meisler & Midyette (1994)	Manager Clinician Consultant Educator Researcher
Taylor (1999)	Patient identification/outreach Individual assessment and evaluation Service planning Resource identification Service implementation Care monitoring Advocacy
Stanton *et al.* (2000)	Coordinator Liaison Collaborator Promoter Negotiator Facilitator Evaluator
White (2004)	Assessor Advocate Facilitator and coordinator of care Planner Monitor
Evercare (2004)	Champion Clinician Communicator Coach Care orchestrator

Competency Framework

In 2006 the Department of Health produced an educational framework for community matrons and case managers following the NHS Modernisation Agency and Skills for Health (2005), a collaboration on a community matrons competency framework. The framework has been published to provide guidance on raising the standards of health and social care by supporting healthcare professionals to develop appropriate knowledge and skills needed for case management. The education framework states that community matrons will need to develop competency in all nine domains (see *Table 5.2*) while the case manager who does not provide advanced nursing care will have to achieve competency in eight domains. The competencies set out in domain A reflect the NMC competencies for advanced practice. Community matrons will have to demonstrate this through Masters level practice, but they will not need a full Masters degree (DH 2006). The level at which the case manager will perform case management will depend on the complexity of the caseload for which they are responsible – this will be set by the employing authority (DH 2006).

Although the Department of Health (2006) has stated the domains are essential for community matrons and case managers they are not exclusive as other competencies need to be considered, for example, cultural diversity, information technology and clinical governance.

Table 5.2 Community matrons and case managers competency framework (DH 2006)

	Domains
A	Advanced clinical nursing practice*
B	Leading complex care coordination
C	Proactively manage complex long-term conditions
D	Managing cognitive impairment and mental well being
E	Supporting self care, self management and enabling independence
F	Professional practice and leadership
G	Identifying high-risk patients, promoting health, preventing ill health
H	Managing care at the end of life
I	Interagency and partnership working

* not applicable to case managers

Interprofessional Working

Following the 1990 Community Care Act, case management was used for providing care for frail older people. The case managers were trained social workers (Murphy 2004) and their target client group was the same as those thought to be suitable for community matrons. This has now been expanded to incorporate other healthcare professionals as identified by the NHS and Skills for Health (2005). This supports work already undertaken by Kaiser Permanente who used experienced medical social workers and nurses (Bodenheimer 2002b). Robbins and Birmingham (2005) have highlighted a gap in the relationships between nurses and social workers, identifying the following reasons:

- Ownership of case management, which led to issues around job security
- Lack of understanding about what each profession does, and the type of work each professional undertakes.
-

For case management to work, it is important for health professionals to work towards a more interprofessional relationship (Evercare (2004); Yamishita *et al.* 2005). However, the workforce needs to develop the skills that allow them to share power and work in teams (WHO 2004).

Case management is both disciplinary and interdisciplinary. Individuals have adopted and practised case management but no discipline owns it (Huber 2002). If there is no collaboration between the disciplines, confusion occurs as to what case management is.

Tribalism

According to Hunter (1996) all developed healthcare systems operate on the basis of tribalism, where managers, nurses and professionals allied to medicine are composed of various tribes. Each tribe has different goals and perceptions of what constitutes effective care, so they pull in different directions. Community matrons and case managers will need to work across boundaries and build networks to promote change using negotiation if they are to work collaboratively (DH 2006). For interprofessional working to be effective, cooperation and collaboration are essential (Rushmer 2005).

Informally, staff are asked to blur boundaries to reduce rigid role and care provision demarcations, but this can cause ineffective interprofessional working. Tasks would not be clearly defined and health and social care professionals would not know who was providing the care, resulting in ambiguity and misunderstanding (Rushmer 2005). For effective interprofessional working, there is a sharing of tasks, skills, knowledge, attitudes and interest.

Partnership Working

Case managers also need to consider their partnership working with patients. They need to include patients in decision-making in all aspects of their healthcare (WHO 2004). To do this case managers need the skills to share power and involve patients. They need to be able to:

- Communicate well
- Negotiate and share decisions
- Solve problems collectively
- Establish joint goals
- Implement action
- Identify strengths/weaknesses in care packages
- Clarify roles and responsibilities
- Jointly evaluate programmes of care.

Information Technology

The introduction of case managers has made a difference to many people's lives, but case managers have to trawl through paper databases to identify people at risk (Dr Foster Intelligence 2006). Accessing informative databases will help case managers:

- Identify people at risk
- Track the effectiveness of their care
- Track patient outcomes, cost and quality.
-

Predicting who is most at risk is a complex but essential role of the case manager (WHO 2004). Patients at risk of re-hospitalisation (PARR) was developed using hospital episode statistics (NHS 2005). It is essential that all healthcare professionals have ongoing training in the use of information systems to make proper diagnoses for treatment management.

Evaluation of the Role

Gravelle *et al.* (2006) stated that community matrons are likely to be popular with patients and increase access to care but they are unlikely to reduce hospital admissions, unless there is a more radical design system. Lillyman and Saxon (2007) stated that community matrons can provide anecdotal evidence from patients and local statistical evidence that there is a need for the role, but research needs to be undertaken on the effectiveness of the role. A postal survey of 119 community sisters, general practitioners and practice managers carried out by Armour (2007) identified that 68% were clear about the role and 83% found working with community matrons increased their understanding of the role. However, Armour (2007) states that it is only a small survey and that further research is required on the role.

For case management to continually expand and be effective, ongoing performance evaluations of the case manager role and the programmes of care should be undertaken (Hutt *et al.* 2004). These will help to identify areas for further development (Peterson 2004). Pre- and post-evaluation studies are essential with all new roles, as they assist with future planning (NHS 2005).

Conclusion

Community matrons and case managers have an important role working at the interface between primary and secondary care, ensuring that people with long-term conditions receive appropriate and timely care. There is a need to clarify the roles and their impact on providing care. These roles need to be researched and evaluated and the findings widely disseminated.

References

(all websites accessed 6 March 2008)

Armour J (2007) Early perceptions of the role of community matrons. *Nursing Times* **103**(23): 32–33

Audit Scotland (2005) *Managing people with long-term conditions.* Performance Audit Study

B (1979) Role theory: Expectations, identities and behaviours. New York, Academic Press. In Schmitt N (2005) Role transition from care giver to care manager, Part 1. *Lippincott's Case Management* **10**(6): 294–302

Bodenheimer T, Long K, Holman H *et al.* (2002a) Patient self management of chronic disease in primary care. *Journal of the American Medical Association* **288**(19): 2269–2475

Bodenheimer T, Wagner E, Grambach K (2002b) Improving primary care for patients with chronic illness. *Journal of the American Medical Association* **288**(14): 1775–1779

Bodenheimer T, Long K, Holman H *et al.* (2002a) Patient self management of chronic disease in primary care. *Journal of the American Medical Association* **288**(19): 2269–2475

Bodenheimer T, Wagner E, Grambach K (2002b) Improving primary care for patients with chronic illness. *Journal of the American Medical Association* **288**(14): 1775–1779

Beardshaw V, Towell D. (1990) *Assessment and case management: implications for the implementation of 'Caring for People'.* The King's Fund Briefing Paper 10. Kings Fund, London

Colyer H (2004) The construction and development of health professionals: where will it end? *Journal of Advanced Nursing* **48**: 406–412

Cudney AE (2002) Case management: a serious solution for serious issues. *Journal of*

Healthcare Management **47**: 149–153

Department of Health (1990) *National Health Service and Community Care Act*. London, HMSO

Department of Health (2002) *Chronic disease management and self care. A practical aid to implementation in primary care*. London, The Stationery Office

Department of Health (2004) *NHS Improvement Plan. Putting people at the heart of public services*. London, The Stationery Office

Department of Health(2005a) *Supporting people with long-term conditions: NHS and social Care Model to support local innovation and integration*. London, The Stationery Office

Department of Health (2005b) *Long-term conditions Information Strategy: Supporting the national service framework for long-term conditions*. London, The Stationery Office

Department of Health (2006) *Caring for people with long-term conditions: an education framework for community nurses and case managers*. Leeds, DH

Dr Foster Intelligence (2006) *Keeping people out of hospital: the challenge of reducing emergency admissions*. London, Imperial College

Drennan V, Goodman C, Leyshon S (2005) *Supporting experienced hospital nurses to move into community matron roles*. The Primary Care Nursing Research Unit (www.ucl.ac.uk/pcps/research/pcnru)

Evans C, Drennan V, Roberts J (2005) Practice nurses and older people: a case management approach to care. *Journal of Advanced Nursing* **51**(4): 343–352

Evercare (2004) Implementing the Evercare Programme: Interim Report (www.natpact.nhs.uk/cms/186.php)

Gravelle H, Dusheiko M, Sheaff R *et al*. (2007) Impact of case management (Evercare) on frail elderly patients: controlled before and after analysis of quantitative outcome data. *British Medical Journal* **334:** 31–34

Handy C (1993) *Understanding Organizations* (4th edn). London, Penguin

Harrell H, McCulloch S (1986) The role of the clinical nurse specialist. *Journal of Nursing Administration* **16**(10): 44–48

Huber D (2002) The diversity of case management models. *Lippincott's Case Management* **7**: 212–220

Hunter D (1996) The changing roles of healthcare personnel in health and healthcare management. *Social Science and Medicine* **43**(50): 799–808

Hutt R, Rosen R, McCauley J (2004) *Case managing long-term conditions. What impact does it have on older people?* London, The King's Fund

Kane RL, Flood S, Bershadsky B *et al*.(2003) The effect of Evercare on hospital use. *Journal of the American Geriatric Society* **51**(10): 1427–1434

Lillyman S, Saxon A (2007) Much more research is needed before we write off community matrons. *Nursing Times* **103**(21): 12

Long MJ (2002) Case management model or case manager type? That is the question. *The Health Care Manager* **20**: 53–66

Lyon JC (1993) Models of nursing care delivery and case management definitions of terms. *Nursing Economics* **11**(3): 163–178

Meisler N, Midyette P (1994) CNS to case manager: broadening the scope. *Nursing Management* **25**: 44–46

Murphy E (2004) Case management and community matrons for long-term conditions. *British Medical Journal* **329**: 1251–1252

NHS Modernisation Agency and Skills for Health (2005) *Case Management Competencies Framework: for the care of people with long-term conditions*. London, Department of Health

NHS National Workforce Projects (2005) Long-term conditions. Workforce Development

Pack. Manchester, NHS Workforce Projects. (www.healthcareworkforce.nhs.uk)

Oda D (1977) Specialised role development: A three-phase process. *Nursing Outlook* **25**(6): 374–377

Owen M (2006) An important perspective on the case manager role. *Lippincott's Case Management* **11**: 2–3

Peterson V (2004) When quality management meets case management. *Lippincott's Case Management* **9**(2): 108–109

Plant R (1987) *Managing Change and Making it Stick*. Glasgow, Fontana

Pruitt SD, Epping-Jordan JE (2005) Preparing the 21st century global healthcare workforce. *British Medical Journal* **330** :637–639

Reimanis C, Cohen EL, Redman R (2001) Nurse case manager role attributes: fifteen years of evidence-based literature. *Lippincott's Case Management* **6**(6): 230–239

Robbins C, Birmingham J (2005) The social worker and nurse roles in case management. Applying the Three Rs. *Lippincott's Case Management* **10**(3):120–127

Rushmer R (2005) Blurred boundaries damage inter-professional working. *Nurse Researcher* **12**(3): 74–85

Schmitt N (2005) Role transition from caregiver to case manager, Part 1. *Lippincott's Case Management* **10**(6): 294–302

Slack M, McEwen M (1999) The impact of interdisciplinary case management on client outcomes. *Family and Community Health* **22**: 30–49

Spilsbury K, Meyer J (2001) Defining the nursing contribution to patient outcome: lessons from a review of the literature examining nursing outcomes, skill mix and changing roles. *Journal of Clinical Nursing* **10**(10): 3–14

Staines R (2007) Community matron levels way off target. *Nursing Times* **103**(19): 9

Stanton M, Walizer E, Graham J *et al.* (2000) Case management: a case study. *Nursing Case Management* **5**: 37–45

Stanton M, Dunkin J (2002) Rural case management nursing role variations. *Lippincott's Case Management* **7:** 48–55

Stanton M, Swanson M, Sherrod R *et al.* (2005) Case management evolution: from basic to advanced practice role. *Lippincott's Case Management* **10**: 274–284

Taylor P (1999) Comprehensive nursing case management: an advanced practice model. *Nursing Case Management* **4**(1): 2–13

Vere-Jones E (2007) Government plays the numbers game. *Nursing Times* **103**(19): 8–9

Weiss M (1998) Case management as a tool for clinical integration. *Advanced Practice Nursing Quarterly* **4**: 9–15

White A (2004) Case management and the national quality agenda. Partnering to improve the quality of care. *Lippincott's Case Management* **9**(3): 132–140

Williamson GR, Webb C, Abelson-Mitchell N *et al.* (2005) Change on the horizon: issues and concerns of neophyte advanced healthcare practitioners. *Journal of Clinical Nursing* **15**: 1091–1098

World Health Organization (2002) *Innovative care for Chronic Conditions – Building Blocks for Action. Global report.* Geneva, WHO

World Health Organization (2004) *World Health Report: Changing History.* Geneva, WHO

Yamashita M, Forchuk C, Mound B (2005) Nurse case management: negotiating care together with a developing relationship. *Perspectives in Psychiatric Care* **41**: 62–70

Zander K (2002) Nursing case management in the 21st century: intervening where margin meets mission. *Nursing Administration Quarterly* **26**: 58–68

CHAPTER 6

Pushing the boundaries

Sarah Knight

The need for effective management of patients with long-term conditions has been highlighted as a priority in the *NHS Improvement Plan* (DH 2004). This forms a core element of national service frameworks and has been at the forefront of the political agenda with an emphasis on developing the community matron/case management (CM) role in order to promote this service. The RCN document *The Future Nurse* (2004) discussed challenges that the health and social care system would give us over the next decade. It discussed the need for an appropriately trained workforce to meet the demands of these expectations, to avoid issues around stress and sickness.

Many projects have specifically examined the CM role and how this needs to be developed to mirror the philosophy and vision of the new NHS. For example, the report on the Evercare Project (2003) lists critical new initiatives for which that project has been a catalyst. With the Department of Health (2006) challenging the paternalistic approach to healthcare and promoting the belief that users should exercise choice and opinions about care they receive, CMs will be at the forefront of care delivery for many of these patients.

This chapter explores the skills required to develop the role of the CM. Throughout the chapter professional accountability and the independent practitioner will be addressed.

Leadership and Collaboration Skills

Northouse (2004) defines leadership as a 'process' in order to achieve a common goal. Castledine and McGee (2003) state that leadership qualities for advanced nurses are instrumental in encouraging collaboration, as one person can hardly ever meet all the needs of patients. Within the CM arena it has been difficult to promote true collaborative practice due to different philosophies of care adopted by various professions. The SWOT analysis (Iles & Sutherland 2001) shows that leadership and collaborative practice are lacking in many areas (*Table 6.1*). This role provides an opportunity to help develop the CM's practice to provide a more seamless service. For example, general practitioners (GPs) may be reluctant to

Table 6.1 SWOT analysis

Strengths	**Weaknesses**
Wide knowledge base within the team The new team gives me the opportunity to develop Experience gained invaluable Training available to develop service Motivated team Many ideas within team to share knowledge	Lack of protocols and pathways Lack of advanced skills Time limited Lack of knowledge from other professionals about the role lack of collaboration from wider members of the team Some poor communication Inadequate leadership skills to try and prevent these weaknesses
Opportunities	**Threats**
I can develop my own skills and contribute to the development of the role Training opportunities Experience that goes alongside new role Government policy is supporting case management	The need to meet targets and fears Expectations of others to meet certain criteria Others do not want to relinquish parts of their new role Information technology — the need to keep up-to-date The need to prove cost effective

share patients' notes without written consent from management level, and social inclusion staff tend to conduct their own assessments, which may omit joint assessments. Conlon (1997) stated that the issue around confidentiality can hamper collaboration due to the differing ways people work.

When working with specialist nurses the case manager has noted that they are reluctant to 'give up' certain roles to provide a more seamless service, citing that they are experts within that field and that passing over part of their role may lower standards. Castledine and McGee (2003) state that while collaboration and multidisciplinary working are essential, ultimately each member of the team is personally accountable for their own actions, and the law does not recognise a lowering of standards when activities are undertaken by nurses rather than doctors.

Case Manager's Role in Promoting Collaboration

The need for the CM to promote effective collaboration within areas of practice stems from the use of good leadership and communication skills (Rossi 2003). A report from the Evercare model (2003) and its lessons also demonstrates the need for effective collaboration in proactive generalists rather than reactive specialists to create a ripple effect that calls forth positive responses from the team in understanding the value and practice of care collaboration. It is clear that if the CM is at the centre of care management, he/she should take responsibility for developing collaborative relationships between primary and secondary care resources for highly complex patients (Matrix Research and Consultancy 2004).

The CM has to build on skills such as open communication, assertiveness, negotiation and coordination, which are seen as an essential part of collaborative practice (Wells *et al.* 1998). They also have to develop the ability to share problems — and Hanson *et al.* (2000) suggest that this is the main skill in promoting good collaborative care.

Communication Skills

In reviewing the current position of a case manager gaps have been identified. It had been noted that the leadership and collaboration aspects of this role require development and communication skills. By formalising these it was possible to develop an action plan that clarifies differences and focuses on complementary approaches to achieve common goals. Rossi (2003) says that these are key elements to achieve true collaboration and the formalisation of practice is what has been missing from the case manager's current practice. To do this, she says, is to build on current skills by stating clear visions with all members of the team with upfront agreements about roles and decision making, which in turn builds trust. However, to achieve this, some professionals may envisage giving up some of the 'power' that they perceive is theirs. This, say Kouzes and Posner (2002), is wrongheaded and inconsistent with all the evidence on high-performing organisations, and can ultimately result in conflict and resistance.

Advanced Clinical Practice

The advanced health assessment element of the case manager's role requires the most development, with the opportunity to practise advanced health assessment within the workplace being seen as an essential element (Castledine & McGee 2003). It is identified in the SWOT as both a weakness and an opportunity. The skills outlined within the leadership element of development also play an essential part within advanced practice because the case manager needs to:

- Engage in critical analysis of patient care and outcomes
- Provide information to challenge the *status quo*
- Work effectively within the organisation (Castledine & McGee 2003).

Competencies for the Case Manager

The skills required to develop advanced practice can be difficult to conceptualise as coined by Schon (1983), who placed a high value on intuition and the ability to draw on practice experiences. Schon advocated the use of an epistemology of practice. However for the CM a comparison between current competence levels, and competence levels as stipulated by Skills for Health (2005), is useful. Rossi (2003) states that this approach is effective if the job description:

- Is clear
- Delineates the responsibilities and functions of the case manager
- Reflects the expectations and level of education of the case manager.

The need to develop the skills from those of general nursing knowledge to those of advanced and independent practitioner is more than just learning these skills We also need to acknowledge that the CM will practise at a level with much more autonomy and responsibility (Hickey *et al.* 1996).

Critical Thinking

Although the CM is developing good advanced assessment skills, true advanced practice is more than just this. Therefore the CM needs to focus on a critical approach to the assessment and not rely heavily on written text, but question and challenge normal practice. Critical thinking within the health assessment is, according to Castledine and McGee (2003), essential to support clinical judgments and decision-making, facilitating the development of 'intellectual independence and relativistic reasoning', so that the CM thinks like a clinician as well as a nurse. The skills required for the CM to develop to reach this point include:

- In-depth reading
- Receiving feedback from mentors

- Forming groups where clinical judgments can be questioned in a positive arena
- Presenting patients' stories to groups
- Working collaboratively with all members of the team.

Rossi (2003) discusses the use of protocols as being imperative in developing the clinical role of the CM. This area for development for the CM is seen as vital as it directs, monitors, and evaluates treatment and outcomes and can support issues surrounding accountability.

Marketing the Service to other Professionals

A gap in the CM's skill, and also a weakness as identified in the SWOT analysis, is the ability to sell the service using market forces. GPs and other professionals are still undecided as to the benefit of case management, and it is the initial implementation stage and the benefit incurred which is hoped will alter their mind set. The biggest challenge is getting other professionals to accept the benefit of the CM role and relinquish some of their responsibilities.

It has been easy for the CM to carry on providing a service to the patients and dealing with problems as they arise without addressing the bigger issue that the service needs marketing and people's attitudes need changing. Paton and McCalman (2000) suggest that it is an easy route to ignore problems such as this in the hope that performance can be maintained, but say that in today's climate the human element cannot be ignored as part of the change process. Brooks and Brown (2002) suggest that the negativity a role can create is quite often preserved by an organisation, and to maximise value for money and effectiveness we have to change our practice which will feed into a wider organisational change.

Creating Capacity for Change

The interim report from the Evercare project (2003) discusses the initiatives into the NHS and talks about the CM's capability of achieving transformational change. The ability to change the practice of those around the case manager to incorporate their service within everyday planning is underway but has reached a stop due to resources and time available. Harding (2004) suggests that the next step forward is for the CM to create the capacity for change and then action it. He suggests that the CM needs to use information, intuition, ideas and instincts necessary to implement the change of practice before implementing the marketing process to change other professionals' ways of working. In order to do this, he says the CM needs to monitor and analyse data and have the ability to keep everyone informed. Paton and McCalman (2000) say that to act as the change agent the person (the CM) will need to describe him/herself, the problem and what is going on and essentially have the ability to apply a descriptive-analytical capability combined with the skill of diagnosis. Buchanan and Huczynski (1997) identified that the key competence for managing a change was the ability to handle it, and Buchanan and Boddy (1992) identified key skills – communication, motivation, facilitation and knowledge.

Changing people's practice to incorporate the case management process means there are going to be barriers. Kanter (1983) points out that many people say 'yes' to a change initially but then when impact begins a host of negative comments and actions materialise. The resistance to changing practice is not uncommon, and Paton and McCalman (2000) suggest that this is because people fear the unknown and are comforted by the familiar. It is clear that a certain amount of 'tribalism' is apparent within some roles in the CM arena and it has been a weakness of the CM to break down the barriers. These are the skills that need to be developed and Wakley and Chambers (2005) state that these skills are based around the person being a good change agent.

Professional Accountability for Independent Practice

Skills for Health competencies (2005) set out what is required for the CM and the expectations for practice, with pressure to undertake this role at the end of formal training. However, we have to accept that it is the personal and professional responsibility of the CM to ensure the work is within the scope of professional practice and to refuse to undertake activities outside competence levels.

Accountability, according to Tingle (1995), has various definitions and starting points depending on which angle you take. For example McSherry and Pearce (2002) consider accountability as being concerned with changing practice. Dowling *et al.* (1996) looked at accountability as being obligations arising from professional regulations, being accountable for our actions and being answerable to them. The NMC *Code of Professional Conduct* (2002) says being accountable is being:

> *'...responsible for something or to someone'.*
>
> *NMC (2002)*

This refers to being answerable for your actions and omissions, and accountable for promoting the interests and dignity of all patients. We must also acknowledge our limitations. Being an independent practitioner within the role of a CM is no defense if newly appointed and feeling the need to carry out tasks – the CM should expect training in the same way that patients should expect competent practice (DH 1996).

The World Health Organization identifies the healthcare organisation as responsible for providing training for healthcare workers that goes beyond acute skills in order to support the management of chronic conditions. The CM should be aware of evidence-based guidelines for the treatment of these conditions (WHO 2002).

The need for the CM to consider accountability in addition to previous practice is because the role has expanded to cover complex issues surrounding independent practice. Collaboration and multidisciplinary working, although essential for the case manager, can have an impact on the issues surrounding accountability as ultimately each member of the team is personally accountable for their own actions.

Using Protocols

A research study conducted by the RCN (2004) suggests that when issues of accountability arise the use of protocols were of value. Within independent practice the CM has to act within boundaries of competence and can insist on specialist training (Castledine & McGee 2003). They too value the use of protocols for use during independent practice.

For the CM the use of protocols for independent practice may be the most useful way to ensure accountable practice using intuition by deviating from the protocol when needed by the use of a 'variance'. 'Variance' and 'variance tracking' allow the professional to deviate from a pathway if there is a valid reason (Shuttleworth 2003). Shuttleworth says that the benefits of using protocols or integrated care pathways extend to the patient, the practitioner and the service provider. She also states that they can improve issues outlined above, such as collaboration, decision making, and marketing.

McCollom and Allison (2004) discussed the use of clinical practice guidelines around the issue of accountability for independent practice. They said that guidelines can help the CM to make decisions about appropriate healthcare in certain situations, and can be flexible, with deviations acceptable.

Theoretical Frameworks

More specific to case management, the Council for Case Management Accountability (CCMA) has been developing standardised performance measurements for case management (Howe 2005). This outlines a theoretical framework for performance, measurement and improvement in outcome measures. This again goes some way in introducing standardised practice for advancing practice to include collaboration, implementation, etc., and help ensure quality of care delivery.

For the CM to be accountable to the stakeholders they serve is imperative, as according to Rossi (2003) doing the right thing at the right time and for the right reason ensures the trust relationship that is the foundation of case management. The CM in practice can help ensure accountability issues are addressed for independent practice by:

- Developing the skills outlined above
- Ensuring competence levels are maintained
- Using resources such as protocols and integrated care pathways.

Conclusion

It is clear that case management throughout the country is at different stages of development and that learning from good practice is vital. Castledine and McGee (2003) recognise that advanced practice creates a challenge to nurses to creatively express values, knowledge and skills in uncharted territory. The CM maintains that we can do this by identifying areas for development and within support systems we can create an improved service for all. It is clear that by developing the CM role we are being given opportunities of which early generations of nurses may only have dreamed, and in the CM arena it seems that we can develop higher-level skills to allow the practitioner to function in a different way. One way is by giving us the ability to identify areas for development and action plan their progress.

References

(all websites accessed 6 March 2008)

Brooks I, Brown R (2002) The role of ritualistic ceremonial in removing barriers between subcultures in the National Health Service. *Journal of Advanced Nursing* **38**(4): 341–352

Buchanan D, Boddy D (1992) *The Expertise of the Change Agent.* London, Prentice-Hall

Buchanan D, Huczynski A (1997) *Organisational Behavior: an introductory text* (3rd edn). London, Prentice-Hall

Castledine G, McGee P (2003) *Advanced Nursing Practice* (2nd edn). Oxford, Blackwell Publishing

Conlon M (1997) *The Hub in Bristol.* Unpublished workshop paper presented at the Homeless and Roofless Conference, Birmingham, July.

Department of Health (1996) Risk Management in the NHS. London, NHSME

Department of Health (2004) *NHS Improvement Plan: putting people at the heart of public services*. London, DH

Dowling S, Martin R, Skidmore P *et al.* (1996) Nurses taking on junior doctors' work: a confusion of accountability. *British Medical Journal* **312:** 1211–1214

Evercare (2003) Implementing the Evercare Programme: interim report. (www.natpact.nhs.uk)

Hanson C, Spross J, Carr D (2000) Collaboration. In: Hamric A, Spross J, Hanson C (eds) *Advanced Nursing Practice: an integrative approach,* 315–347. Philadelphia, WB Saunders

Harding P (2004) *Managing Change: a guide to how to manage change in an organization.* Envirowise & Government Office for the South West

Hickey J, Ouimette R, Venegoni S (1996) *Advanced Practice Nursing.* New York, Lippincott

Howe R (2005) Performance measurement for case management: principles and objectives for developing standard measures *The Case Manager* **16**(5): 52–56

Iles V, Sutherland K (2001) *Organisational Change. A review for healthcare managers, professionals and researchers.* National Coordinating Centre for NHS

Kanter R (1983) *The Change Masters: Corporate Entrepreneurs at Work.* New York, Thomson

Kouzes JM, Posner BZ (2002) *The Leadership Challenge.* San Francisco, Jossey-Bass

Matrix Research and Consultancy (2004) *Learning Distillation of Chronic Disease Management Programmes in the UK.* London, Modernisation Agency

McCollom P, Allison L (2004) Clinical practice guidelines: a tool for case managers. *The Case Manager* **15**(4): 5053

McSherry R, Pearce P (eds) (2002) *Clinical Governance: a guide to implementation for healthcare professionals.* Oxford, Blackwell Science

Northouse P (2004) *Leadership: Theory and Practice.* London, Sage Publications

Nursing and Midwifery Council (2002) *Code of Professional Conduct: standards for conduct, performance and ethics.* London, NMC

Paton R, McCalman J (2000) *Change Management. a guide to effective implementation.* London, Sage Publications

Rossi PA (2003) *Case Management in Health Care.* Philadelphia, Elsevier Science

Royal College of Nursing (2004) The Future Nurse: a vision. London, RCN Institute.

Schon D (1983) *The Reflective Practitioner: how professionals think in action.* London, Avebury

Shuttleworth A (2003) *Protocol-based Care.* London, Emap Healthcare Ltd.

Skills for Health/SQW (2005) *Assessing Education and Training Provision for the Health Sector* (Sector Skills Agreement Stage 2). Bristol: Skills for Health.

Tingle J (1995) *The Legal Accountability of the Nurse. Accountability in Nursing Practice.* London, Chapman & Hall

Wakley G, Chambers R (2005) *Chronic Disease Management in Primary Care.* Oxford, Radcliffe Publishing Ltd

Wells N, Johnson R, Salyer S (1998) Interdisciplinary collaboration. *Clinical Nurse Specialist* **12**(4): 161–168

World Health Organization (2002) *Innovative Care for Chronic Conditions: Building Blocks for Action.* Geneva, WHO

CHAPTER 7

Support networks for the case manager/ community matron

Sue Lillyman and Ann Saxon

We all need time to reflect and be supported in our practice — and this is especially important and valuable to those undertaking new roles in professional practice. For community matrons and case managers, who also work in isolation, support and time to reflect may be particularly difficult to access. In this chapter we review some of the ways community matrons and case managers can access support that will help them not only with their demanding role but in developing as advanced practitioners and in pushing their role boundaries forward.

We describe some of the approaches we have used with case managers and community matrons that have helped them to fulfil their own continuing professional developmental needs, maintain their knowledge and skills dimensions (DH 2006) while offering support to and from other colleagues who are also new to the role.

Time to Reflect

We all require some time to think about and reflect on our practice, but finding that time can be difficult. The contribution to role development through reflection has been well documented over the last few decades (Burnard 1988, Coutts-Jarman 1993, Ghaye & Lillyman 2006). Support is important for practitioners — to provide care we also need to be cared for in a secure environment as well as developing our own practice. However, with a busy schedule and working in isolation the workplace environment in the community is not conducive to a supportive reflective environment. The community matron and case manager need to find time to meet with others to gain that support and find time to reflect to develop their practice.

When delivering a postgraduate certificate for the newly appointed community matrons and case managers, we found that one of their main concerns on completion of the programme was assessing support from their colleagues once they were back on their own in practice. The practitioners need to identify the value of support and make time to meet with others.

Purpose of a Supportive Framework

The value of reflective practice for the professional development has been well recorded and most practitioners see the value of it once they start receiving some form of support (Lillyman 2006). However, when working in isolation there is little time for reflection and little incentive to take time out to reflect. Those who do take time to reflect without support may find reflection less effective if they have limited personal knowledge of the area of practice or if they over-reflect — which in itself can be dangerous. The values of reflecting with others are:

- Support gained from spending time with colleagues
- Wider knowledge-base of the group when reviewing the issues raised
- Guidance of other colleagues in the reflective process.

Support can help the practitioner to:

- Be more self-aware and help to improve care (Taylor 2001)
- Enhance accountability and promote professional development (Clouder & Sellars 2004)
- Improve competences and skills (Rundgvist & Severinsson 1999).

Setting up a Supportive Network

In the West Midlands, the first cohort of case managers and community matrons accessing a postgraduate programme found that they had developed as a group throughout the course. They were afraid of losing that rich source of support and development when the course came to an end. To continue this support, the group decided to form its own networking forum. They met three to four times a year and gained sponsorship for a venue. During their meetings they invited a guest speaker to discuss up-to-date policies and developments within the NHS, so including an educational aspect to the event. One of the most valuable aspects of this meeting was the networking they were able to continue with colleagues and the opportunity to discuss practices across the primary care trusts. Time was allowed for this to take place both informally over a meal and formally in the group session, sharing ideas and group work. The sharing of practice and developments helped people to feel less isolated and review current trends within their own area of practice. As the role has developed within different primary care trusts they were able to share these, identify changes and areas of practice that had benefited from those changes as well as those that had been less successful.

Setting up and running the forum did, however, require commitment from the community matrons and case managers in practice as the meetings were held in the evening and required people to attend following work. A steering group was also formed with representatives from across the West Midlands area and members from the university so that the meetings could be planned and relevant speakers invited to take part. All the community matrons and case managers were invited to take part and these were not limited to those who had attended the course.

Action Learning Set

Other forms of support the case managers found particularly useful was the action learning set approach developed for management education in the 1970s (Pedler *et al.* 2005). Some community matrons and case managers felt that they wanted something that was more local and based within their own trust.

Action learning sets were introduced into the healthcare arena by the Royal College of Nursing through their leadership programmes (Royal College of Nursing 2002). The action set involves a group of six to eight professionals who meet on a regular basis to listen, question, challenge and action plan areas of practice (Lillyman 2007). Through this process the community matrons and case managers can support each other in decision-making and problem-solving as well as developing new skills. The difference between this approach and the more traditional group clinical supervision approach is that the group do not offer advice to their peers. In action learning sets the person bringing an issue shares this within the group, who then offer supportive and challenging questioning that leads the person presenting to form their own action plan.

Lewin (1963) noted that a person who makes their own decisions is more motivated than a passive target of other people's views. The Royal College of Nursing (2002) suggests there are three levels of learning through this approach. People in the group learn about:

- Themselves
- Issues they are tackling within the set
- The process of learning.

During the action learning set an action plan is developed which the practitioner implements into practice. At the next meeting, the consequences of the actions are fed back to the whole group so that they can learn from the way this was played out in practice. The sessions are based on reflection,

Models for Action Learning

When starting the action learning set it can be difficult for practitioners to adopt the challenging and probing questions. For this there are several models that can be used by the group to guide the questioning. These models include:

- Six Honest Serving Men (Kipling 1902)
- Force field analysis (Lewin 1963)
- Mind mapping (Buzan 1993) (Ghaye & Lillyman 2006)
- Six Thinking Hats (de Bono 2004)
- Five Whys (Senge *et al.* 1994)
- SWOT analysis (Rogers 1999)
- Z techniques (Rogers 1999)
- Perceptual positioning (RCN 1996)
- Six Shoes (de Bono 1996)
- Six Value Medals (de Bono 2005)

Each model has a slightly different approach to supporting the group through the questioning process and helps to guide the focus of the questioning. If they are not used to this type of questioning, the group needs to decide which approach will be used rather than attempting an eclectic approach.

problem solving and decision making in a supportive environment.

A facilitator may or may not be present in the session. However, one person needs to take responsibility for timekeeping, allowing the presenter to present their issue and guide the group in their questions. As many healthcare practitioners are used to problem solving there is often the temptation to revert to providing advice to the presenter. The group needs to adopt the Rogerian approach of probing and questioning while offering support (Rogers 1999) during these sessions.

The community matrons and case managers have valued the action set approach, as opposed to the more clinical supervision approach, as they feel this allows them to develop as practitioners and make their own decisions and action plans in a supportive environment.

Clinical Supervision

The more traditional approach to support can be obtained through clinical supervision. However, we note that there is no single clear definition of clinical supervision (Davey *et al.* 2006). With the introduction of the Health Care Standards set out by the Department of Health (2006), clinical supervision for healthcare workers has found itself back on the agenda. With confusion about the process and the lack of uptake by practitioners in the nursing field, many trusts are now referring to this process as 'practice support' to remove the concept of a hierarchical and surveillance process of supervision in the workplace that is often misinterpreted through the title. (Peniket & Lillyman 2007).

There have been a number of approaches to clinical supervision models and practitioners should use the one with which they feel most comfortable and can access.

Case managers and community matrons may be more familiar with clinical supervision than with action learning sets. With supervision they have the option of using the one-to-one approach, group supervision or networking. The practitioner can still gain support in their own development and again the approach is based on reflecting on their practice and developing new ways of working and expanding the boundaries. They may choose a group approach where six to eight practitioners meet to discuss issues. Here one of the group takes on the role of supervisor to support and guide the group. They may prefer a one-to-one session where they meet together and ones take on the role of supervisee and the other of supervisor.

If the practitioner is unable to meet with others and wishes to use a wider networking approach, they can access this through their own network as noted above or through the NHS community matrons network (www.networks.nhs.uk). This website has discussion forums for practitioners to use as support and reflection with other practitioners.

Choosing a Model of Support

We have mentioned several approaches to gaining support that the case manager and community matron can access. It is really down to the practitioners and their preference which approach they use. The important issue is that they gain that support through and with their colleagues.

Meeting KSF/Professional Body Requirements

Practitioners do not have to do all the above to fulfil their professional development, Department of Health Standards (DH 2006) and their personal professional plans. The practitioner can gain all their professional requirements though one of the approaches. The trust for which the community matron or case manager works needs to be notified of the event and method – but not the content – of the discussion, to meet its own standards.

To meet their professional requirements, the community matron and case manager need to keep their own personal records and reflections from the action learning set or clinical supervision session. With this they can identify their continuing professional development for any professional body's requirements, i.e. *Nursing and Midwifery Professional Portfolio* (NMC 2004), *Knowledge and Skills Frameworks* domains (DH 2004) or any other developmental plan's requirements for the individual performance reviews. If the practitioner maintains their records from the sessions they can produce these for all the above without having to repeat the reflections or try to gain professional development through several routes.

Conclusion

Community matrons and case managers need to continue to support each other in their current practice, development and continuation of the role. They need to take time out for that reflection and support of each other.

References

Burnard P (1988) The journal as an assessment and evaluation tool in nurse education. *Nurse Education Today* **8:** 105–107

Buzan T (1995) *The Mind Map Book.* London, BBC Books

Clouder L, Sellars J (2004) Reflective practice and clinical supervision: an interprofessional perspective. *Journal of Advanced Nursing* **46**(3): 262–269

Coutts-Jarman J (1993) Using reflection and experience in nurse education. *British Journal of Nursing* **2**(1): 77–80

Davey B, Desousa C, Robinson S *et al.* (2006) The Policy-Practice Divide – who has clinical supervision in nursing? *Journal of Research in Nursing* **11**(3): 237–248

de Bono E (1996) *Six Action Shoes.* London, HarperCollins

de Bono E (2004) *How to have a Beautiful Mind.* London, Vermilion

de Bono E (2005) *The Six Value Medals.* London, Vermilion

Department of Health (2004) *The NHS Knowledge and Skills Framework (NHS KSF) and the Development Review Process.* London, DH

Department of Health (2006) *Standards for Better Health.* London, DH

Ghaye T, Lillyman S (2006) *Learning Journals and Critical Incidents* (2nd edn). Dinton, Quay Books

Kipling R (1902) *Just So Stories.* Latest edition, London, Walker Books, 2004

Lewin K (1963) *Field Theory in Social Science: Selected Theoretical Papers.* London, Tavistock Publishing Ltd

Lillyman S (2006) Practice support (clinical supervision) survey of staff report January 2006. Unpublished report. Birmingham, SBPCT.

Lillyman S (2007) Action learning sets and clinical supervision. In Lillyman S, Ghaye T.

Effective Clinical Supervision: The Role of Reflection (2nd edn). Dinton, Quay Books

Nursing and Midwifery Council (2004) *The PREP Handbook*. London, NMC

Pedler M, Burgoyne J, Brook C (2005) What has action learning learnt to become? *Action Learning Research and Practice* **2**(1): 49–68

Rogers J (1999) Facilitating groups. London. Management Futures Ltd

Royal College of Nursing (1996) Nursing Leadership – Study Guide. London. RCN

Peniket D, Lillyman S (2007) Implementing clinical supervision within a primary care trust. In Lillyman S, Ghaye T (eds.) *Effective Clinical Supervision: The Role of Reflection* (2nd edn). Dinton, Quay Books

Rogers J (1999) *Facilitating Groups*. London, Management Futures

Royal College of Nursing (1996) *Nursing Leadership – Study Guide*. London, RCN

Royal College of Nursing (2002) *Facilitators Toolkit: techniques for action learning sets*. RCN Clinical Leadership Team. London, RCN

Rundgvist EM, Severinsson EI (1999) Caring relationships with patients suffering from dementia – an interview study. *Journal of Advanced Nursing* **29:** 800–807

Senge P, Kleiner A, Roberts C *et al.* (1994) *The Fifth Discipline Field Book: strategies and tools for building a learning organization*. London, Nicholas Brealey

Taylor (2001) *Reflective Practice: A Guide for Nurses and Midwives* (2nd edn). Milton Keynes, Open University Press

Index

F

G

H

I

K

L

M

N

P

Q

R

S

T

W